Disclaimer

The Care Code is provided for general educational and informational purposes only. It does not provide medical, legal, financial, or caregiving advice and it should not be relied upon as a substitute for guidance from qualified, licensed professionals.

Nothing in this book is intended to diagnose, treat, cure, prevent or manage any disease, condition, injury or health-related issue. Always consult a physician, licensed healthcare provider, attorney or other qualified professional regarding medical conditions, medications, care plans, legal matters or major decisions affecting health, safety or well-being. Never delay or disregard professional advice because of information contained in this book.

Caregiving situations, health conditions and outcomes vary widely from person to person. What works for one individual may not be appropriate or safe for another. The strategies, examples, worksheets, exercises, checklists or tools discussed in this book are general in nature and may not be suitable for every reader or circumstance.

Any references to technology, digital tools, artificial intelligence (AI), predictive systems, reminders or supportive resources are provided for educational awareness only. These tools are not guarantees of safety, health improvement, independence, prevention of hospitalization or any specific outcome.

By reading and using this book, you understand and agree that you are solely responsible for your decisions and actions. You assume all risks associated with the use or misuse of the information provided and that no physician-patient, caregiver-client, fiduciary or professional relationship is created.

The author and publisher make no guarantees, representations or warranties, express or implied about the accuracy, completeness, reliability or results of using the information in this book.

To the fullest extent permitted by law, the author and publisher disclaim all liability for any loss, injury, damage, or adverse outcome whether direct, indirect, incidental or consequential arising from the use of or reliance on this book.

The images in this book are illustrative depictions designed to strengthen the message of The Care Code. While some are inspired by real experiences, the individuals shown are not intended to represent actual people.

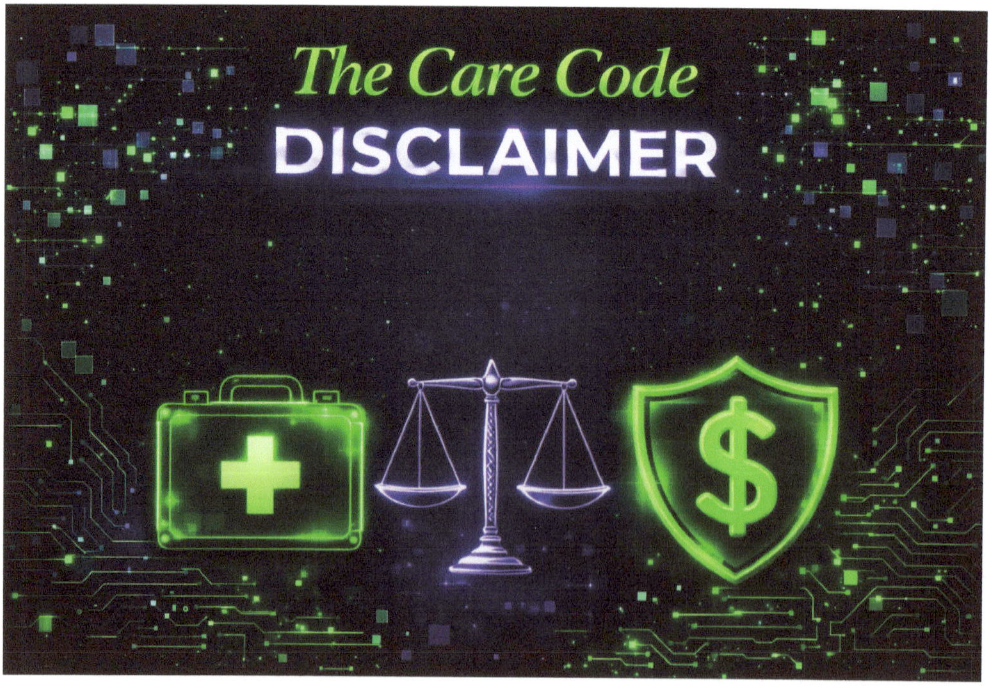

THE CARE CODE

Where PREVENTION Meets AI

Unlock the secrets through love, action, AI technology & intention

Editors: Latric Campfield-Brown, Marrissa Campfield-Kenion
Copy Editor: Scott Johnson
Contributing Editor: Dr. Indira Minus-Grimes , Family Medicine and Gerontology Specialist
Interior Layout and design: Krysten McCartney
Publisher: Senior Living Consultants, LLC
Address: 254 Chapman Rd, Ste 208, #7500 Newark, DE 19702
Phone: +1 954.610.3732
Copyright Year: 2026
ISBN: 979-8-9904070-1-5

Printed in the United States of America

Dedication

The Care Code is dedicated to two individuals whose lives revealed both the urgency, humanity and the heart behind this work. The Care Code is dedicated to my mother-in-law, Kathryn Johnson, who we lovingly refer to as "Mam Mam".

In mid-2024, Mam Mam suffered a fall that changed everything. What followed was a series of hospitalizations and rehabilitation stays that revealed how quickly independence can be lost when care is reactive instead of preventive. Before her fall, Mam Mam, at 82 years old, was still working as a caregiver herself. She was independent, purposeful and full of life. One moment altered her health span and her future, reminding us how fragile aging can be.

This book is also dedicated to Burt Firtel, founder of Remember2, Inc., whose vision inspired the creation of an early-warning health intelligence platform. At 86 years old, Burt experienced what many older adults quietly endure forgetting daily tasks, suffering multiple falls and feeling invisible in moments when he needed to be seen. His concern that others were feeling the same vulnerability became the catalyst for building a system rooted in dignity, prevention and foresight.

Your journey opened our eyes to what caring truly means. Because of you, we learned that care must begin before crisis, when the first quiet signals appear and there is still time to protect what matters most. This book is our promise to do better, to listen sooner, act earlier and care more intentionally. May your story inspire others to protect the dignity, independence and precious moments of those they love.

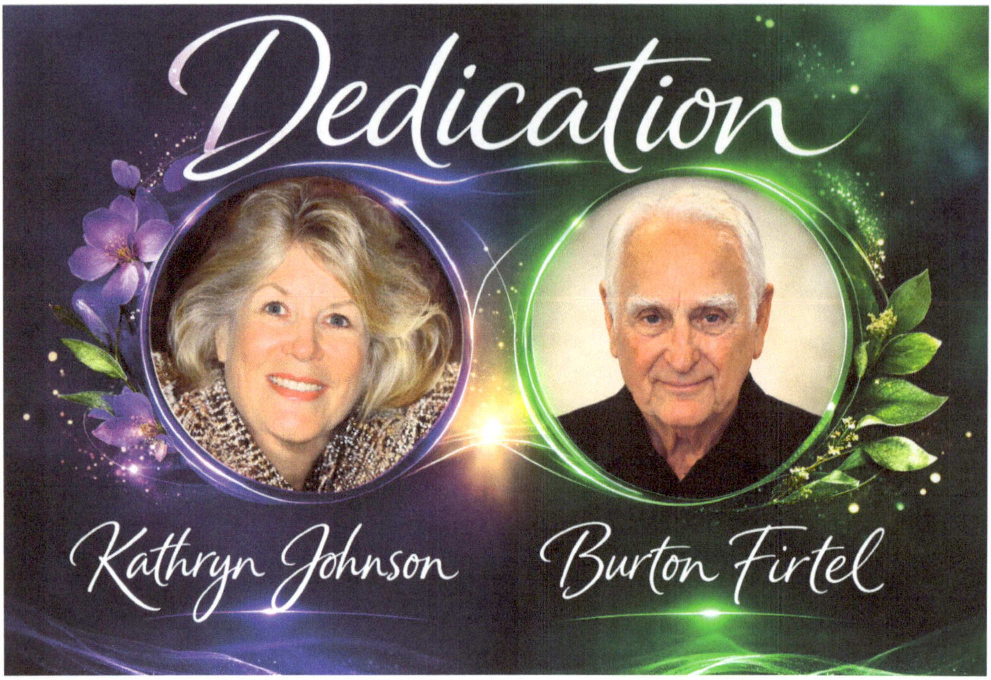
Dedication
Kathryn Johnson
Burton Firtel

Foreword

By Dr. Michelle C. Powell, DO, MPH
Powell Health Solutions, LLC

As a physician, I have spent my career caring for people at some of the most vulnerable moments of their lives. I have seen fear, hope and heartbreak, often all in the same day. I have also seen a troubling pattern repeat itself far too often: care that arrives only after a crisis has already occurred.

Most medical emergencies do not come out of nowhere. They build quietly. Blood pressure rises unnoticed. Oxygen levels dip subtly. Stress accumulates. Fatigue becomes normalized. Families and caregivers do their best, yet without visibility into what is happening beneath the surface, they are left reacting instead of preventing. The Care Code exists because that model is no longer sufficient it speaks to a truth clinicians understand well but rarely say plainly, what we see on the outside is not always a true reflection of what is happening inside the body. A person can look "fine" while their physiology tells a very different story. By the time symptoms become obvious, opportunities for early, simpler intervention may already be lost.

As a practicing physician, I believe deeply in care that is proactive, compassionate and grounded in insight. Prevention is not about fear. It is about awareness. It is about giving families, caregivers and individuals the tools to recognize early signals, ask better questions and act with intention rather than urgency.

What makes The Care Code important is that it does not ask technology to replace human judgment or connection. Instead, it places intelligence alongside compassion, recognizes the emotional toll of caregiving, the reality of burnout and the need for boundaries that protect both the caregiver and caretaker.

This book also acknowledges something many families struggle to face and that is caring for someone, especially as they age. There are moments that test our limits and force difficult decisions. The Care Code meets those moments with honesty, dignity and guidance.

As medicine continues to evolve, so must the way we think about care. Tools like continuous monitoring and early-warning systems, when used thoughtfully, can support healthier outcomes not just for patients, but for families and caregivers. They provide another layer of awareness, one that helps us intervene earlier, communicate better and reduce avoidable harm.

I commend Corlette Deveaux for creating a work that is both courageous and practical. The Care Code invites us to move beyond reactive care and toward a more intentional, informed and humane approach, one that respects life, healthspan and the people who carry the responsibility of care.

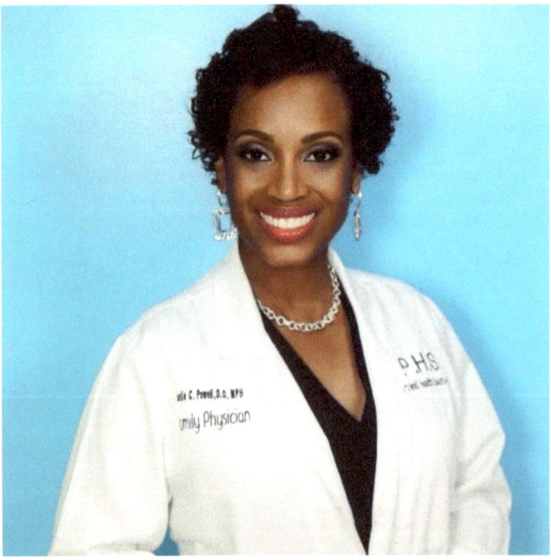

Dr. Michelle C. Powell, DO, MPH
Powell Health Solutions, LLC

The Care Code Pledge

"True Care does not wait for the fall, it watches, protects and acts while there is still time."
- Dr. Regina Marranzini, MD, AGSF

"My husband's journey with sickle cell has taught us to trust God and pay attention to the signals of health. Faith sustains us and tools like Rm2.ai give us continuous visibility into his vital signs so we can act before a crisis"
- Wanda McPhee, Caregiver and Wife

"When I suffered a stroke, I realized the signal Rm2.ai detected the day before wasn't just data, it was a warning that contributed to saving my life."
- Scott Johnson, MS

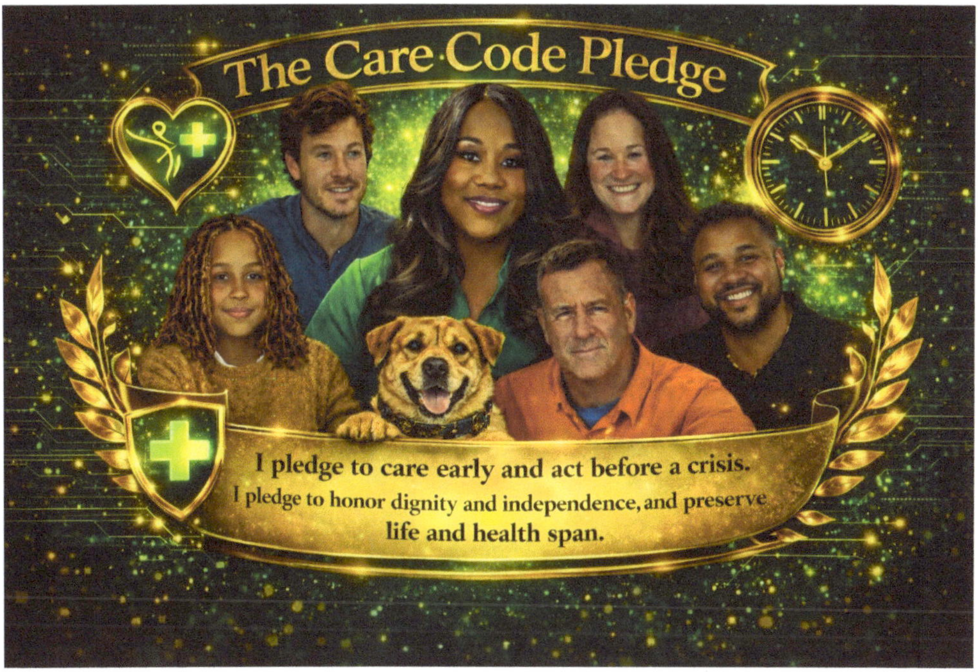
The Care Code Pledge
I pledge to care early and act before a crisis.
I pledge to honor dignity and independence, and preserve life and health span.

Preface

No one expects a fall to change everything. It happens quietly in a kitchen, a bathroom, a familiar hallway. One small moment, and life is divided into before and after. Before, there is independence and strength. After, there are hospital rooms, uncertainty and questions no family feels prepared to answer.

In mid-2024, my family experienced this firsthand. My mother-in-law, an active 82-year-old, suffered a fall that set off a cascade of hospitalizations and worsening chronic conditions. What we later realized was that there had been earlier warning signs. The issue was not a lack of love or medical care, it was a lack of early detection. Care began after the crisis.

The Care Code was born from a simple belief: prevention is the highest form of care. When subtle changes in mobility, vital signs, hydration, medication adherence or engagement are recognized early, intervention becomes possible. Dignity can certainly be preserved. Decline can be slowed. Outcomes can be improved.

This book is not about replacing human care. It is about strengthening it, equipping families, caregivers and healthcare professionals with insight so they can act sooner, not later. Aging does not have to be defined by crisis. With foresight, connection and compassion, it can be supported with intention.

Welcome to The Care Code. The future of care begins before the fall or crisis.

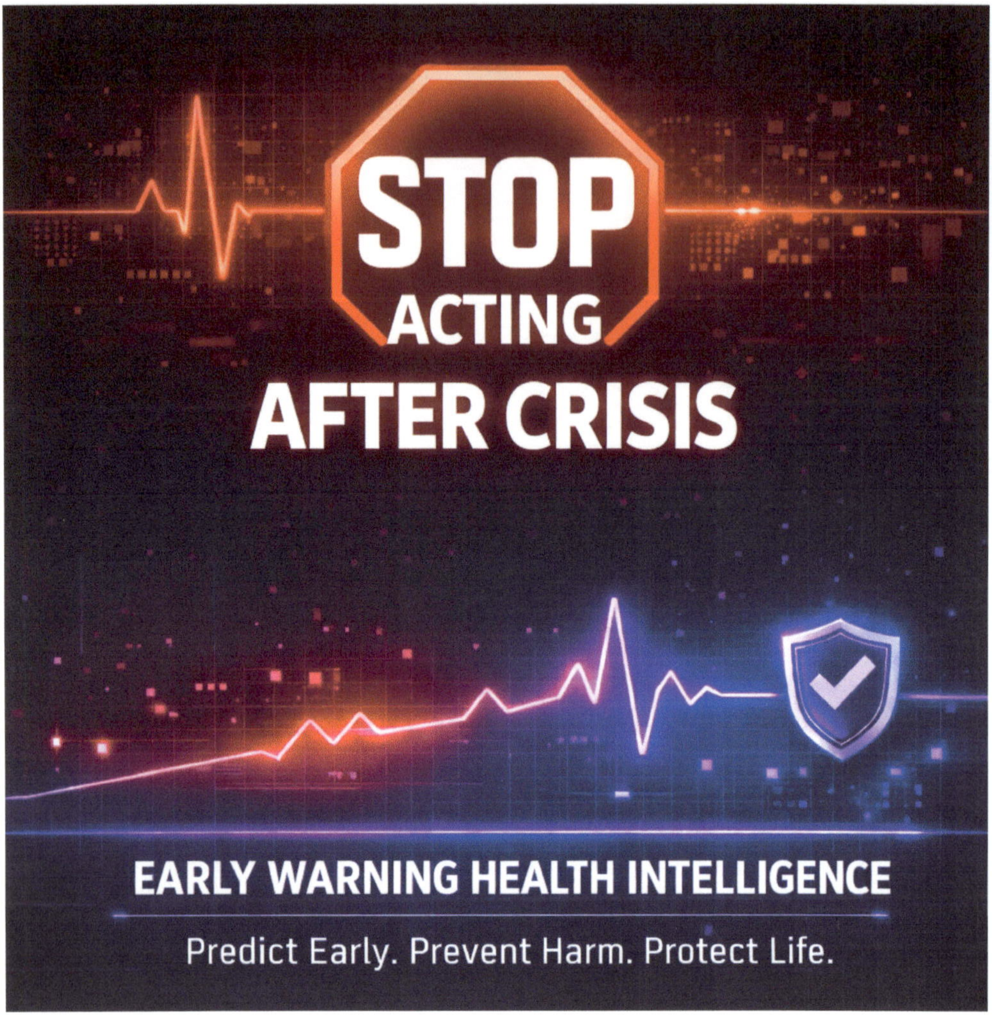
STOP
ACTING
AFTER CRISIS
EARLY WARNING HEALTH INTELLIGENCE
Predict Early. Prevent Harm. Protect Life.

Table of Contents

Introduction

Cracking The Code

Imagine a world where a loved one's fall, missed medication or potential health crisis does not spiral into an emergency. Where caregivers, families and healthcare providers have eyes, ears and insight CONTINUOUSLY, anticipating health issues before they happen. In the past, this could have been science fiction, but no more. Artificial Intelligence (AI), Rm2.ai™ is now leading the charge to crack the "Care Code".

Every year, 1 in 4 adults over 65 experiences a fall, leading to over three million emergency room visits and one million hospitalizations annually (CDC, 2024). Millions more face preventable complications from missed medications, dehydration, wandering and infections, costing the US healthcare system hundreds of billions and cutting years off life and health span for many (CDC; PubMed, 2024). The Care Code exists essentially to minimize these statistics and increase overall quality of care.

Sadly, I have personal experience with an unanticipated medical crisis. In 2021, my mother, Eunice Deveaux, suffered a stroke because her hypertension was not being managed. She was not adhering to the medical protocols shared by her physicians. Unfortunately, this resulted in a stroke, hospitalization and she ultimately passed away on September 24, 2021. This mirrors the experiences of millions of families worldwide.

Traditional care systems, though well-intentioned, cannot monitor every moment or detect subtle patterns that precede crises. But AI-powered platforms, like Rm2.ai™ can. Through continuous monitoring, real-time data, predictive analytics and automatic intelligent alerts, we can decode the signals our loved ones' bodies and behaviors are sending, possibly before danger strikes. Even something as simple as a reminder to take medication can prevent a life-altering event.

The Care Code is a roadmap for a new era of care. Inside, you'll find eye-opening statistics that expose the true scope and cost of today's health care crisis, alongside practical, real-world strategies for thoughtfully integrating AI into caregiving, strategies designed to protect independence, preserve healthspan and uphold dignity. At the end of the book, thought-provoking games invite you to pause, reflect and apply what you learned.

At the conclusion, you will understand that caring smarter isn't a future possibility, it's here. Because care is not reactive. It is about action and it is intentional. And it begins by cracking the code.

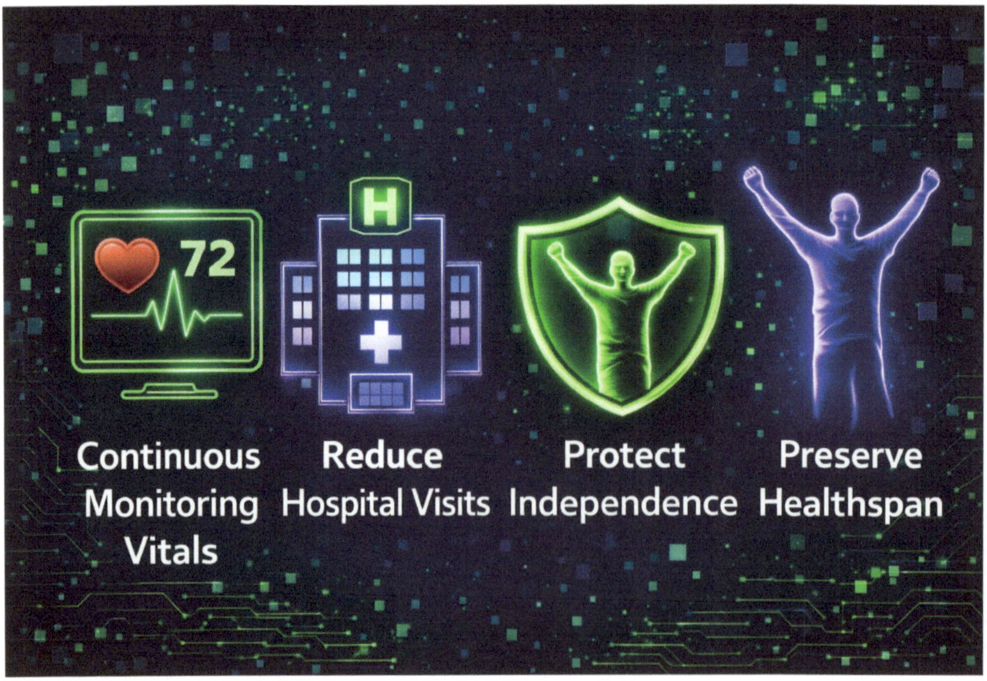

1

Why Health Care Needs Innovation

Every year, millions of seniors face risks that are preventable, yet too often overlooked. In the United States alone, more than 14 million adults age 65 and older fall each year. Falls are the leading cause of fatal and nonfatal injuries in this age group. About 3 million emergency department visits and 1 million hospitalizations stem from older adult falls annually, with tens of thousands of deaths (CDC, 2026). Falls can restrict activity, shorten lifespan, cause disability severely impact quality of life or worse cause death.

Falls are just one part of a larger problem. Medication non-adherence, when people do not take prescriptions as directed, creates its own cascade of risk. This contributes to disease progression, preventable hospitalizations and billions in avoidable healthcare costs. Approximately 40 – 50 % of older adults do not take medications properly and an estimated 10 – 30 % of hospital admissions in seniors are linked to adverse drug reactions or misuse (World Health Organization, 2003). Medication non-adherence, dehydration, falls and elopement cost our healthcare system and families hundreds of billions each year, highlighting the urgent need for preventive, proactive care.

At the same time, the world is aging faster than ever. This demographic shift will place unprecedented strain on families, caregivers and health systems worldwide. By 2030, 1 in 6 people on the planet will be age 60 or older and by 2050 the global population aged 60+ is projected to double to 2.1 billion.

Consider Eunice, a 78-year-old grandmother who cherished her independence.

Her family worried constantly, but daily monitoring was impossible. One afternoon, a few missed doses of her blood pressure medication led to a mild stroke, a fall and hospitalization. An incident, in a different health ecosystem, might have been prevented with predictive technology and timely reminders. Data shows that "low medication adherence may be associated with an increased rate of falls among older adults." (NIH, 2022).

Eunice's story is deeply personal because she is my mother. Unfortunately, this is painfully common. Every preventable fall, every missed medication, every delayed response represents a loss of independence, escalating healthcare use and emotional strain for families.

Traditional caregiving, though compassionate, is reactive. Families and caregivers often find themselves responding to crises rather than preventing them. Hospitals, insurance companies, organizations and assisted living facilities spend billions every year addressing emergencies that could be mitigated with early warning systems and continuous monitoring, exposing the limits of current health care models.

In the United States, Bahamas, and many other nations, as the proportion of older adults increases, seniors increasingly comprise a significant share of hospital bills. Chronic disease complications and acute events, highlight an urgent need for innovation that supports proactive aging rather than crisis care.

This is where AI enters the picture, to support patient care. Platforms like Rm2.ai™ are not just gadgets, they are lifelines. It continuously monitors vitals, movement patterns, sleep, daily habits and medication adherence. Rm2.ai™ may detect subtle warning signs before a crisis unfolds and will send automatic alerts to caregivers and family. Early evidence from remote monitoring systems shows significant reductions in hospitalizations and emergency visits, shorter hospital stays and lower overall health care costs when health indicators are tracked proactively.

The numbers tell one story but the human impact tells another. Seniors and individuals with chronic diseases retain independence longer and ultimately lives are saved. Families regain peace of mind, because of the Care Code.

The Care Code will show you exactly how this revolution in CARING is happening and how you can unlock its power for your loved ones.

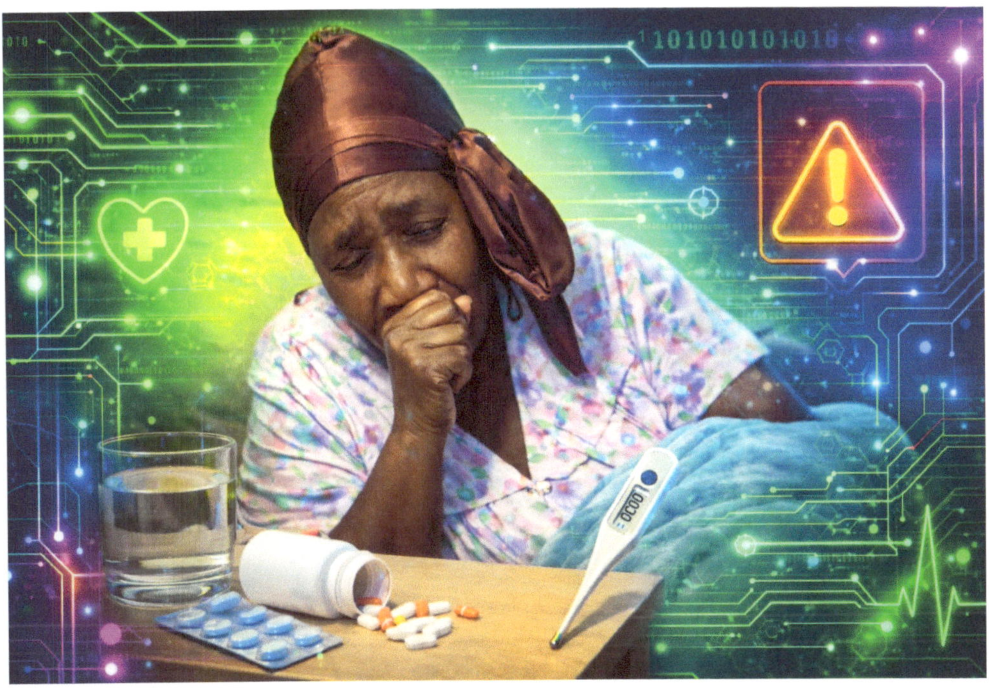

2

The AI Advantage

Technology is often seen as cold, detached or impersonal. But in healthcare especially when it comes to aging and chronic diseases, artificial intelligence is proving to be anything but. Today's AI systems are not futuristic curiosities, they are practical tools with real impact on quality of life, safety and outcomes. AI systems can help detect problems earlier, guide better decisions and alert caregivers before small issues become crises.

At its core, AI shines where the human brain alone cannot. AI systems can sift through thousands of data points every minute, looking for patterns, changes and trends that would otherwise go unnoticed. It does not replace human care, it augments it, amplifying what people are capable of and alerting when action matters most.

For decades, healthcare has been reactive. We wait until symptoms become obvious, until a fall happens, until dehydration escalates or until a lab result is abnormal. AI flips that model on its head. With predictive analytics and continuous monitoring, it can reveal subtle shifts in vitals and behavior before they escalate into emergencies. In assisted living communities, platforms that combine wearables and AI should lead to measurable improvements, lower hospitalization rates and possibly fewer falls. Under continuous AI-supported monitoring, seniors may have longer lengths of residence. (WifiTalents Team, 2025).

This is the future of predictive care, not guessing what might happen, but knowing what is likely to happen next and acting before a crisis occurs.

A new kind of early warning health intelligence system is here. AI excels at recognizing patterns over time. Small changes in activity, such as sleep, gait, heart rate, hydration or behavior may seem insignificant in isolation but together they can tell a story about declining health. Modern AI tools monitor these clues continuously, learning each individual's baseline and alerting caregivers when something deviates from the norm.

This predictive capacity isn't theoretical. AI-driven systems can now detect falls with high accuracy, notify caregivers instantly and even anticipate risk by analyzing gait and movement patterns before an incident happens.

Smarter monitoring equals safer independence. AI doesn't just intervene, it can preserve independence. Health Intelligence, wearable devices and connected sensors can monitor vital signs like heart rate, blood pressure and oxygen levels continuously. They can also detect falls or predict fall risk before it happens, track hydration and behavior changes that signal early health decline. Rather than guesswork, wearable devices support medication adherence with reminders and alerts and personalize recommendations based on real data trends.

These are more than cool features, they are lifesaving tools. They keep seniors living independently longer while giving caregivers the confidence that someone is watching, analyzing and ready to alert when needed.

Beyond safety is enhancing quality of life. The AI advantage goes beyond safety into the realm of daily well-being. Platforms that monitor activity and behavior can encourage routines that support physical, mental, and emotional health like regular exercise, better sleep patterns, and social engagement. These insights bring precision to caregiving, allowing for personalized guidance rather than one-size-fits-all recommendations.

Imagine knowing not just that a parent took their medication, but whenever they skipped a dose, missed a pattern that precedes dehydration or began to move less frequently before a crisis strikes. That is the difference between reaction and prevention.

Let’s be clear, AI does not replace caregivers. It does not replace human love, empathy, intuition or presence. What it does is give caregivers tools they did not have before such as data-backed insights, predictive alerts and continuous monitoring that expand their capacity to care. The human element remains central. The machine simply helps us do more of what matters most with greater precision.

A recent study in The Bahamas, done with the Ministry of Health and Wellness highlights the real-world impact of AI-driven monitoring. Participants in the Rm2.ai™ health Intelligence group experienced zero hospital admissions. Seventy percent of participants in the Rm2.ai group reported fewer health incidents and overall satisfaction with the platform was high. These findings demonstrate the potential of Rm2.ai™ to reduce avoidable medical events, preserve independence and transform caregiving from reactive to proactive.

AI is not cold, it is complementary. It blends machine precision with human compassion. By analyzing what we can not see on our own, it helps us act earlier, protect dignity and preserve health span in a way that was previously impossible.

This is the AI advantage: turning caregiving from reaction into foresight, from crisis management into prevention and from overwhelm into empowered action and intentional care.

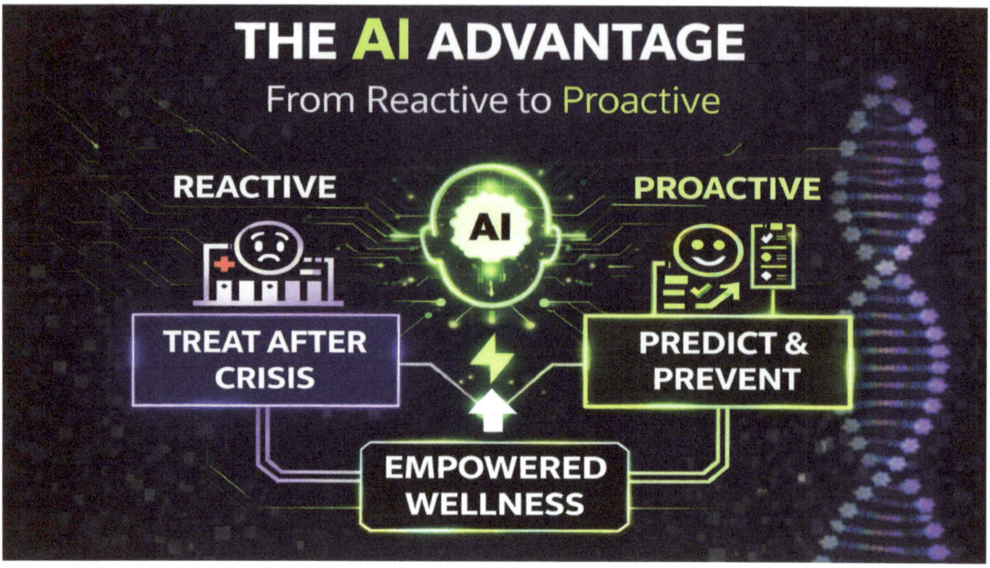
THE AI ADVANTAGE
From Reactive to Proactive
REACTIVE
AI
PROACTIVE
TREAT AFTER CRISIS
PREDICT & PREVENT
EMPOWERED WELLNESS

3

Living Better, Not Just Longer

A longer life means little if those years are filled with preventable suffering, loss of independence and crisis-driven care. How we live may matter more than how long we live. For decades, modern medicine has celebrated a single victory, we are living longer. Advances in antibiotics, surgery, pharmaceuticals and emergency care have pushed average life expectancy to historic highs. On paper, this is a triumph. In reality, it has created one of the greatest paradoxes in healthcare today. We have extended lifespan but too often at the expense of healthspan.

Understanding the difference is important. Lifespan refers to the total number of years a person lives, from birth to death. It measures the quantity of life. On the other hand, health span measures the quality of those years. It is the length of time a person lives in good physical, cognitive, and emotional health, free from disabling chronic diseases, cognitive decline hospitalizations and loss of independence.

This distinction matters because a longer life does not automatically mean a better life. Today, many individuals spend the final 10–20 years of their lives managing multiple chronic conditions, cycling through emergency rooms, juggling medications and relying heavily on family, caregivers or institutional care. Longevity without vitality comes at a high cost financially, emotionally and socially.

There are significant hidden cost of a longer lifespan. When health span lags behind life span the consequences ripple far beyond the individual. Families experience emotional strain, burnout and financial hardship. Additionally, caregivers sacrifice careers, health and stability providers face moral distress and exhaustion. Health systems absorb rising costs from preventable crises and insurers raise premiums to offset avoidable utilization.

Do not overlook the emotional economics of care. The price we pay when decline is managed reactively instead of prevented proactively is astonishing. We are not just adding years to life, we are adding cost, complexity and suffering to those years. It appears that systems may favor lifespan over health span. Why do I believe that lifespan is favored over health span? The current healthcare model is designed to respond to events, not anticipate them. Some reward acute interventions over early detection, crisis management over prevention, treatment after decline rather than protection before it.

Consider this! A fall triggers care, dehydration triggers care, missed medications trigger care, cognitive decline triggers care. Care is triggered after an incident occurs. Unfortunately, by the time care is triggered, damage may have already occurred. Let us replace the reaction triggers to prevention triggers instead. Health span is not extended in emergency rooms. It is preserved in daily life quietly, continuously and proactively.

We have a new measure of success. It is Health span. The future of healthcare demands a new metric of success. Let us shift from the normal standard of care. No longer should the focus be on the amount of procedures performed, how many hospital days were billed or how long someone survived after diagnosis.

Let us develop a new normal where independence is preserved and emergencies are prevented. How much suffering could be avoided and how many families can remain whole and supported, if the norm changed?

Health span reframes care around function, dignity and autonomy. Reframes in health span prioritizes the ability to live safely at home, remain socially connected, manage chronic conditions effectively and age with confidence rather than fear.

There is now an important role of predictive and preventive care. Extending health span requires a fundamental shift from reactive medicine to predictive and preventive care. This is where technology, data and compassionate design converge. By continuously monitoring subtle changes in movement, vitals, cognition, behavior, hydration and medication adherence predictive systems can identify risk before they become a crisis.

A fall prevented may preserve mobility and life span. Increased medication adherence preserves health and early intervention preserves confidence, dignity and time. All combined to support proactive care and preserve life and health span. Health span is not preserved through heroics, it is preserved through early signals and timely action.

A simple Care Code Principle. At the heart of The Care Code is a simple truth: *The goal of care is not merely to help people live longer but to help them live better for as long as possible.*

Extending lifespan without extending healthspan is not progress, it is post-ponement. True innovation lies in protecting the years that matter most. The years when people can still choose, contribute, connect and live on their own terms.

Let's reframe the aged old question. For years, healthcare has asked; "can we afford prevention?" But that is no longer the right question. The real question is: "can we afford the cost of doing nothing?" Every preventable fall, hospitalization and decline shortens health span even if lifespan continues. The Care Code calls for a future where health span becomes the primary goal, the guiding metric and the moral compass of modern care. Because longevity without quality is not a victory. And aging well should not be a privilege, it should be the standard.

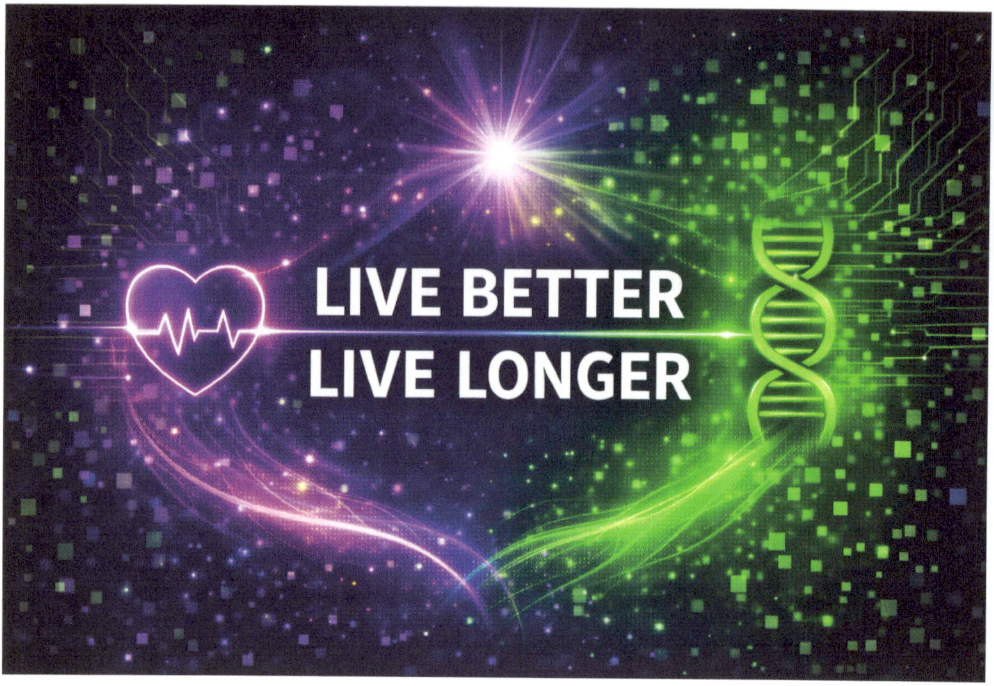
LIVE BETTER
LIVE LONGER

4

The Predictive Power of Data

At the heart of AI-driven care is data; the patterns, signals and insights that tell a story no human eye could see alone. Rm2.ai™ does more than react to emergencies; it predicts them. By analyzing vitals, movement, behavior and routines, it identifies risks before they become crises.

How prediction works. Imagine a senior's daily routine as a complex rhythm. Subtle changes, a slightly slower walk, missed medication, or unusual heart rate fluctuations can signal an impending problem. Rm2.ai™ monitors this data continuously and applies advanced algorithms to detect irregularities. When a pattern indicates risk, the system sends an automatic alert to authorized family members, healthcare providers or caregivers. This early warning capability may be the difference between a minor incident and a life-threatening emergency.

Predictive metrics in action. Rm2.ai™'s patented health intelligence technology continuously monitors multiple factors to provide early insights that may protect health and independence. Rm2.ai™ monitors vital signs such as heart rate, blood pressure, oxygen levels and temperature. At the same time, it supports medication and hydration adherence through reminders, tracking and logging. By analyzing all of these elements together, Rm2.ai™ can detect subtle changes before they become emergencies, enabling proactive, personalized care that may provide peace of mind to families.

The health intelligence platform monitors thresholds and sends automatic alerts when irregularities are identified to prevent avoidable hospital visits.

Predictive data is transforming how care is delivered and more importantly, when it is delivered. Research increasingly shows that when continuous monitoring and AI-driven early warning systems are introduced, outcomes change in measurable meaningful ways. Predictive care shifts intervention upstream, identifying risk before it becomes a crisis.

Multiple studies examining AI-enabled wearable monitoring and remote patient monitoring in older adult populations demonstrate significant reductions in emergency utilization. A meta-analysis published in JMIR reported that continuous monitoring combined with predictive alerts was associated with approximately a 36–38 percent reduction in emergency hospital visits among monitored seniors compared with conventional care. Some intervention groups approaching nearly 40 percent fewer hospital admissions. These reductions are not the result of delayed care, but of earlier, better-timed interventions that prevent escalation altogether.

Falls are one of the most costly and life-altering events in aging and are also increasingly predictable. Research examining AI-enabled gait analysis, motion sensors and activity trend detection shows that fall risk can be identified before impact occurs. Industry-wide analyses indicate that AI-supported monitoring systems can detect falls with 92–99 percent accuracy and are associated with reductions in fall-related identifying risk before it becomes a crisis.

Medication adherence is a major driver of avoidable hospitalizations. It also improves with predictive and reminder-based AI systems. Studies reviewing AI-powered remote patient monitoring in home and senior care settings report improvements in medication adherence ranging from 25 to 40 percent, particularly when reminders, tracking and caregiver alerts are integrated into daily routines. Improved adherence translates directly into better disease control and fewer acute events.

Speed matters in emergencies and predictive systems reduce dangerous delays in care. Automated alerts and real-time monitoring have been shown to cut emergency response times by as much as 50 percent, eliminating the lag between an event and awareness. In care, minutes and sometimes seconds are the difference between recovery and irreversible decline.

These outcomes are not isolated, they reflect broader trends in senior care innovation. The global market for AI in senior care is projected to reach $5.4 billion by 2027, driven by growing evidence that AI tools improve patient safety, clinical decision-making and care coordination while reducing preventable utilization across systems. As adoption grows, predictive care is moving from experimental to essential.

What makes predictive data powerful is not the numbers alone, but how those numbers are translated into action. Visual tools such as risk-score trends, activity heat maps and correlations between vitals and interventions turn abstract data into clear, actionable insight. Families and caregivers no longer have to guess. They can see change as it unfolds and respond with intention.

Traditional caregiving relies heavily on observation, memory and luck. Predictive AI flips that model, and it provides foresight instead of hindsight. This allows caregivers to intervene before emergencies occur. Seniors benefit from safer and longer independence and families gain clarity and peace of mind, with this new model. Care becomes proactive, not reactive.

Ultimately, predictive data does more than prevent crises. It empowers smarter caregiving, preserves dignity, extends independence and improves quality of life. Understanding and using this data is not optional, it is essential. It is one of the keys to unlocking The Care Code.

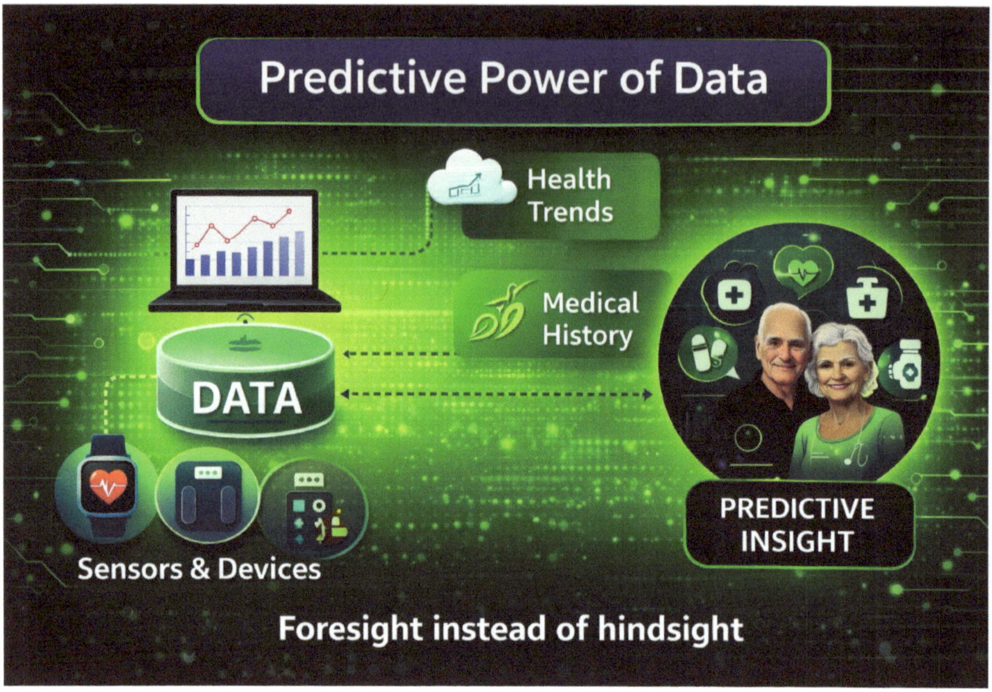
Predictive Power of Data
Health Trends
Medical History
DATA
Sensors & Devices
PREDICTIVE INSIGHT
Foresight instead of hindsight

Did You Know?

Many health crises begin with small warning signs that are often missed or ignored.

Medication Non-Adherence: Many people do not take medications exactly as prescribed. Missed or incorrect doses can quietly worsen chronic conditions.

Dehydration: Even mild dehydration can cause dizziness, weakness, confusion, and increase the risk of falls.

Falls: A fall is often not the beginning of the problem. It can be the result of earlier changes in balance, mobility, medications or overall health.

Chronic Conditions: Most chronic illnesses progress gradually. Small changes in sleep, activity, energy or vital signs may signal that something in the body is changing.

Early Warning: The body sending subtle signals before a crisis occurs.

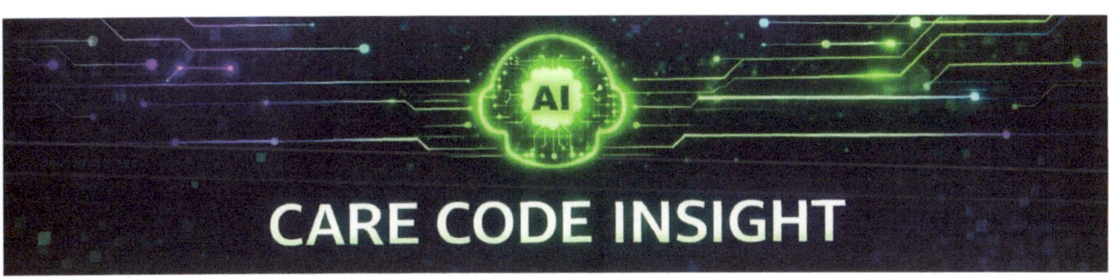

5

Early Warnings Save Lives

Most medical crises do not arrive without notice. They announce themselves quietly through subtle changes that are easy to dismiss, easy to miss and often misunderstood. A missed medication: a restless night, a slower walk, a skipped meal alone, may seem like insignificant signals. Together, these signals tell a powerful story.

The problem is not that families and caregivers do not care. The problem is that the healthcare system has trained us to wait. We are taught to respond when pain becomes unbearable, when symptoms become severe, or when an emergency forces action. By then, damage may have already been done.

Early warnings change everything. Early warning signals are the body's way of asking for attention before it reaches a breaking point. When these signals are recognized early especially through the support of LiveVital Intelligence™ care shifts from reaction to prevention. Falls may be avoided and dehydration, medication non adherence and respiratory decline can be addressed before they become life-threatening.

This is where technology becomes deeply human. AI does not replace caregivers or clinicians. It amplifies their ability to see what the human eye cannot: patterns forming over time. AI connects small data points into meaningful insight, allowing families and providers to intervene early, calmly and confidently. Instead of panic, there is preparation. Instead of a crisis, there is control.

Early warnings also protect dignity. Most seniors do not want to be rescued, they want to be supported. They want to live independently, safely and with confidence. When early signals are addressed promptly, seniors stay in their homes longer, experience fewer hospitalizations and maintain a higher quality of life.

Lives are not only saved in emergency rooms. They are saved in living rooms, kitchens and bedrooms. Particularly when we listen early, act thoughtfully, and care consistently.

Early warnings are not alarms, they are opportunities. And when we respond to them, we unlock one of the most powerful truths in healthcare: PREVENTION. This is the most compassionate form of care.

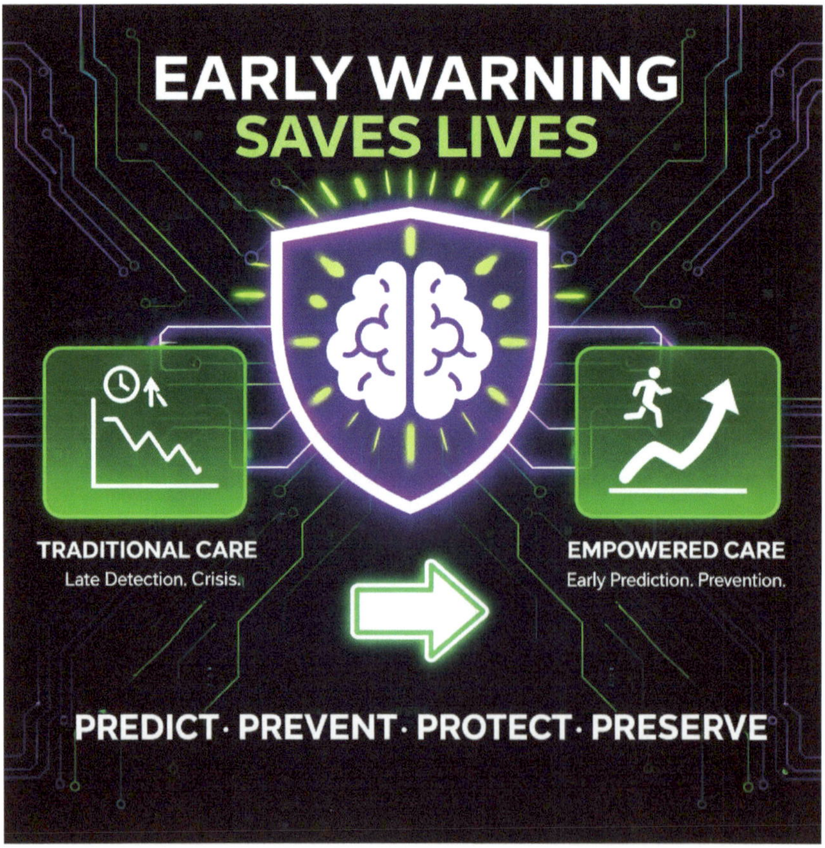
EARLY WARNING
SAVES LIVES
TRADITIONAL CARE
Late Detection. Crisis.
EMPOWERED CARE
Early Prediction. Prevention.
PREDICT · PREVENT · PROTECT · PRESERVE

6

Peppers, Lasagna & Empowerment for Caregivers

Care does not begin in hospitals, it begins at home quietly, daily and often invisibly. Families and caregivers are the backbone of our healthcare system, yet they are rarely given the tools, data or support they need. They are expected to notice everything, remember everything and respond perfectly while balancing jobs, families and their own health. This is not realistic or sustainable.

Empowerment changes the caregiver experience from overwhelming to informed. When families have visibility into what is happening in real time, care becomes proactive instead of reactive. Guesswork is replaced with clarity. Anxiety is replaced with confidence.

Technology when designed with compassion levels the playing field. AI-driven tools allow caregivers to see trends, receive early alerts and act before a situation escalates. This does not remove the human element of care; it strengthens it. Families can focus on presence, connection and love, rather than constant worry.

Empowered caregivers make better decisions, they communicate more effectively with healthcare providers and they intervene earlier. And just as importantly, they protect their own well-being. Burnout is one of the greatest hidden risks in caregiving, often leading to breakdowns in care, unnecessary institutionalization and strained family relationships.

Empowerment also restores dignity to seniors. When caregivers are informed and supported, seniors may experience less disruption, fewer emergencies and more independence. Care becomes something done with them, not to them.

Caregiver burnout is a hidden crisis. Caregivers are the backbone of our healthcare system yet they are often the most overlooked, unsupported and exhausted participants in the care equation. Behind every senior striving to age safely is a family member, friend or caregiver quietly carrying the emotional, physical and mental weight of responsibility.

Caregiver burnout is not a weakness. It is a predictable outcome of prolonged stress, uncertainty and constant vigilance. Studies show that over 60 percent of family caregivers report high levels of emotional stress and more than 40 percent experience depression or anxiety. Unfortunately, burned out caregivers are less able to detect early health changes, increasing the risk of emergencies and hospitalizations. Actually, when caregivers are overwhelmed, everyone suffers, the senior, the family and the healthcare system.

Caregiver burnout often stems from one core issue: reactive care. Caregivers are forced into crisis mode responding to falls, sudden hospitalizations, missed medications or confusing symptoms, without reliable insight into what's happening between doctor visits. They often ask themselves "Is this normal aging or something serious?" or "Am I missing something important?" or "What happens when I am not there?" Sadly, this constant uncertainty creates chronic stress, guilt and fear.

The Care Code supports caregivers too. The Care Code reframes caregiving from constant reaction to informed action. With early warning health intelligence powered by Rm2.ai™, caregivers are no longer expected to "just know" when something is wrong. Instead, they are supported by LiveVital Intelligence™, trend analysis and automatic alerts that may detect risks before exhaustion turns into crisis.

Rm2.ai™ helps caregivers by reducing decision fatigue through clear alerts and insights, sharing the burden across families and care teams, providing visibility of vitals, mobility or routines supporting confidence that they are doing the right thing at the right time. So, caregiving becomes less about constant worry and more about meaningful presence.

Empowered caregivers are not those who do more. They are those who see more clearly. When caregivers have visibility into vital trends, monitoring, medication and hydration adherence they gain the freedom to step back from constant surveillance and step into intentional care. This visibility allows authorized caregivers to sleep better, work without constant fear and be present as family, not just monitors.

While caring for my mother in law, my husband and I started to feel under the weather but yet we pushed forward to care for Mam Mam, who had been in a rehab facility for over 100 days. Knowing that my husband and I weren't feeling well, our friends stepped in. Jacqueline brought stuffed peppers and Ruthe brought lasagna. Meals that nourished our bodies and reminded us that we were not alone. And then there was my dear friend, Dr. Michelle C. Powell, when she heard we were not well, she did not just check in once, she called daily. Dr. Powell asked what we needed and extended herself with intention. She made sure we were supported and on the path to feeling better.

Caregiving can consume you, but The Care Code teaches this: accepting support is not weakness, it's essential. Let others care for you, just as you care for others. Love, meals and kindness from others are fuel for the caregiver's journey. Do not forget that caregivers need support too!

Caring for the Caregiver Is Preventive Care. Supporting caregivers is not optional, it is preventive healthcare. When caregivers are supported, seniors experience fewer emergencies, care quality improves and families remain intact and resilient. The Care Code recognizes a fundamental truth, you cannot protect a life by burning out the person who loves it most.

The future of caregiving is not heroic sacrifice, it is sustainable support. By combining compassion with artificial intelligence, and love with early-warning health intelligence, the Care Code creates a model where caregivers are partners. Caregivers do not become martyrs and families become informed, not fearful. Care is proactive, not exhausting. This is how we care longer, better, and together. The key takeaway is that when you care for others, allow yourself to be cared for too. Your well-being matters too.

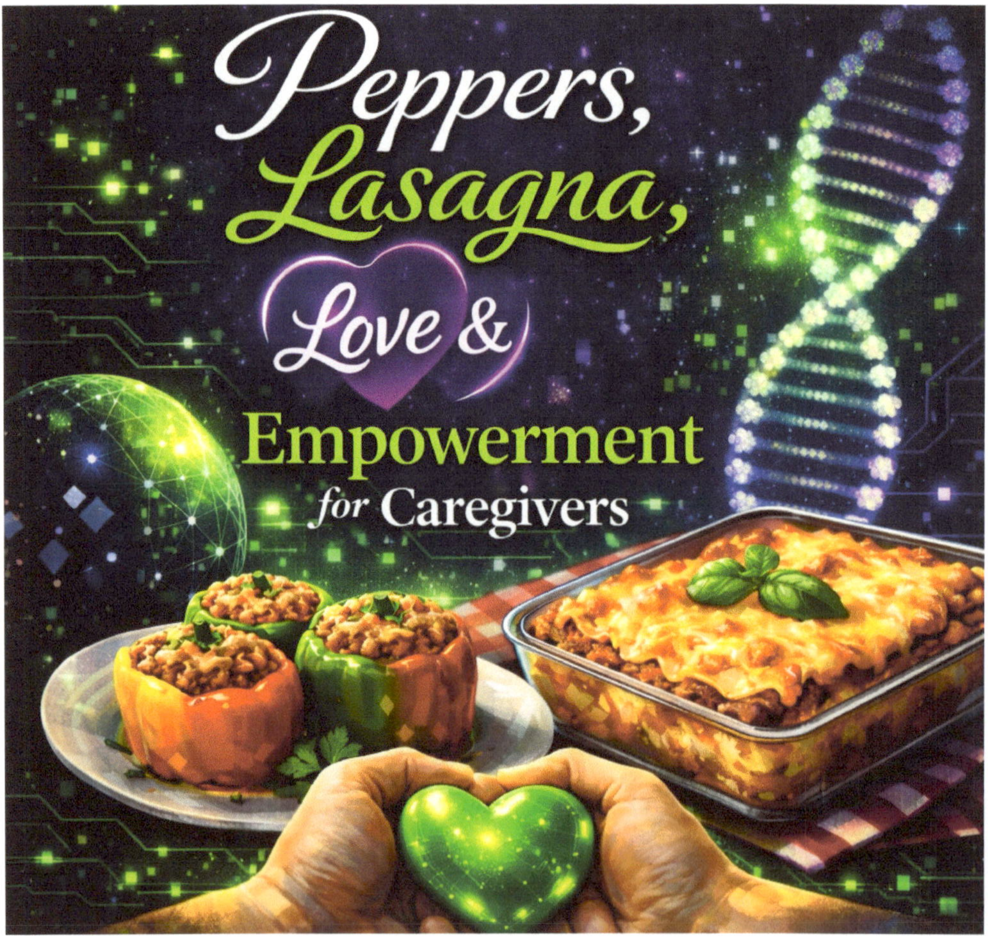

7

The Enema Reality: Caregiving Without Filters

Some of the most important moments in caregiving do not feel important, when they arrive. These moments do not come wrapped in gratitude or recognition. Caregiving does not feel noble or inspiring. They are often awkward, uncomfortable, and deeply personal. And yet, they ask the most honest question of all: Do you really care?

I received a phone call from my mother-in-law from her assisted living facility. Her voice was strained and embarrassed, she was extremely constipated and in pain. She said the facility would not administer an enema, and she needed someone to help her, so she called me. Without hesitation, I told her I would change my plans and come.

Before heading there, I called her daughter and asked if she could meet me at the facility so she could administer the enema. After all, she was her daughter and I was her daughter-in-law. Her response was immediate, she said, "No. I'm not doing that. Why don't you do it?" I gently reminded her that this was her mother. She replied that she was busy, that she might come tomorrow, but that she was not willing to do it. She did not like it and she did not want to. At that moment, I realized this was not about an enema, it was about care. Not the kind of care we talk about. Not the kind we assume comes with a title. But the kind that shows up when something is inconvenient, uncomfortable and unavoidable.

We often confuse caring with what we give, money, gifts or time when it suits us. But caregiving has never been about what feels comfortable or looks generous. It has always been about what needs to be done. True care lives in the spaces most people avoid. Care is not measured by words, intentions or explanations. Care is measured by action.

When we arrived at the facility, my mother-in-law told us she had found someone who was willing to help her with the enema. I felt genuine relief, not because the situation had resolved itself, but because she had been cared for. She deserved care. She deserved kindness. She deserved comfort as she navigated her situation. And once that immediate need was addressed, the quieter needs surfaced, the ones that so often go unnoticed.

Her nails needed to be clipped, so I clipped them. Her clothes needed to be put away, so I folded and organized them. Her room needed to be straightened, so I made it calm and comfortable. I adjusted pillows, checked on her and made sure she felt settled and seen. Beside me, my dear husband was doing the same in his own way, mounting her television, fixing her chair, adjusting what no longer worked and responding to each small request with patience and care. There was no rush, no frustration, no sense of obligation, administering this care, only presence.

Then something unexpected happened. This woman, once strong in stature, independent, decisive, paused. She looked at us and said quietly, "I am grateful. I am grateful for Scott and Corlette." There was no hidden meaning in her words just the truth and genuine appreciation. That moment captured everything The Care Code is about. We were not there to be thanked. We were not there for recognition. We were there because love shows itself in action.

Remember care isn't always pretty. Sometimes it is messy, raw, urgent and deeply uncomfortable. This is the enema reality. My sister, Vonette, is living this with her mother, who is also ill. One day her mother called screaming in pain, begging her to call 911, not because she was dying, but because she was constipated and desperate for relief. The pain was real, the fear was real and their response was care. Vonette and her sister, Dana did not panic or pass it off, they showed up quickly. They got what was needed, and her sister administered the enema that finally brought relief. When it happened again soon after, they did not hesitate, they gave their mother two warm teaspoons of castor oil, easing her pain once more. This is the Care Code in its most honest form and love that rolls up its sleeves. Family that listens to distress and responds without judgment or delay. Care that prioritizes relief, dignity and humanity, no matter how uncomfortable the task.

The Care Code is not about comfort. It is not about preference. It is not about what you like or dislike doing. It is about showing up when someone is vulnerable. It is about choosing compassion over convenience. It is about preserving dignity in the smallest, most human ways.

Care is answering the phone, care is changing your plans and care is doing what needs to be done even when it may be undesirable. And sometimes, care appears to be simple and other times can be profound. Care is also showing up, quietly, when someone needs you most.

This chapter is not about shame or blame. It is about awareness. Because one day, every one of us will need help in ways we cannot control. And when that day comes, the most valuable thing someone can offer us will not be their money, their status or their excuses. It will be their willingness to do the uncomfortable thing with compassion like inserting an enema.

A defining Care Code principle, care isn't about what's convenient, it's about what's necessary. Remember2™ care.

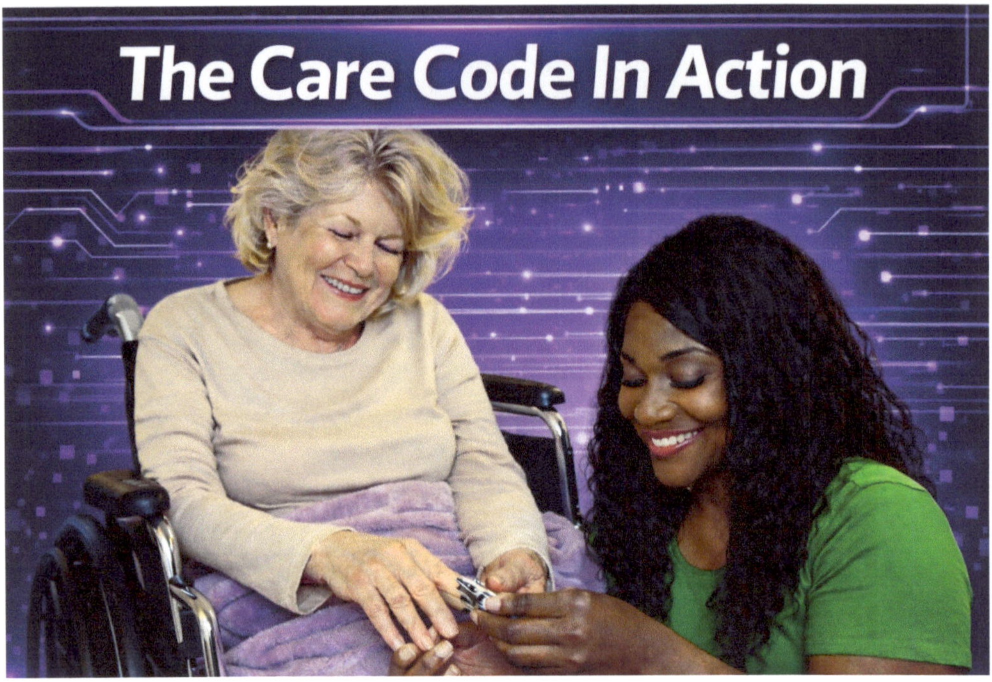
The Care Code In Action

8

Dignity, Independence and Aging in Place

Aging is not a disease. Yet too often, the moment a senior needs support, independence is quickly stripped away. Decisions are made for them instead of with them. Safety becomes the excuse for control. And dignity, the very thing that defines our humanity is unintentionally compromised.

Most seniors want the same thing: to remain in their homes, on their terms for as long as possible. Aging in place is not about avoiding care. It is about receiving the right care at the right time, without sacrificing autonomy, privacy or respect.

The greatest threat to independence is not age, it is uncertainty. Families worry because they don't know what's happening day to day. Caregivers intervene aggressively because they are afraid of missing something. Healthcare systems err on the side of institutionalization because prevention feels risky without visibility.

This is where early warning intelligence and AI-driven insight change everything. When subtle changes are detected early before falls, medication non adherence, dehydration or medical crises, support can be added gradually and thoughtfully. Instead of drastic moves, there are gentle adjustments. Instead of loss of freedom, there is reinforcement of safety. Seniors remain active participants in their own lives, not passive recipients of care.

Technology, when designed with empathy, does more than monitor, it protects. It allows seniors to live freely while ensuring that help is nearby when needed. It reassures families without hovering. This new form of prevention, LiveVital Intelligence™, supports caregivers and providers.

Dignity is preserved when care is invisible, respectful, and timely, aging in place is not a privilege. Aging in place is a right, and with the right tools, insight and compassion. Independence does not have to end when care begins.

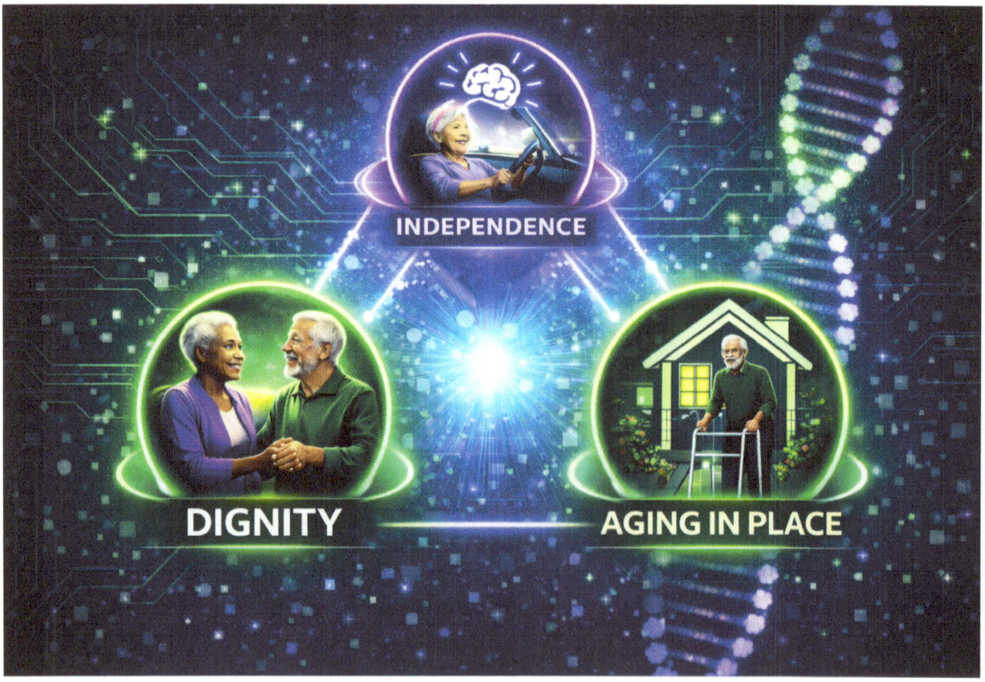

9

Just Listen

Most of us pride ourselves on being strong. We handle things. We carry others and we keep moving, even when life is heavy. But here's the truth: The Care Code reminds us again and again, that even the strongest people need somewhere for their feelings to go.

On January 22, 2026, I felt that quiet weight, the kind that doesn't announce itself loudly but settles into your chest. No, not a crisis, not a breaking point, just anxiety. The kind that comes from watching someone you love struggle and knowing you can not take the pain away.

My husband, Scott, is going through a lot. His mother has been ill for some time. About a year and a half ago, she broke her hip and since then her health has steadily declined. As a result of a fall, she now requires continuous oxygen, has ongoing bed sores along with other physical and cognitive changes. She is experiencing a myriad of emotions including fear, deep anger often expressed through yelling, frustration and emotional outbursts. These emotional outbursts are directed at Scott and her caregivers almost every day.

My mother in law calls my husband constantly for help. Most of the time, she is screaming, ornery or harsh. One day while visiting her, I quietly took her hand, looked her in the eyes and said lovingly, "Mam Mam, can I ask you to do me a huge favor? Can you please stop screaming at my husband and calling him names. He is a great son and husband. When you scream at him, I get the brunt of it at home. Can you be kind to him? We love you and are here to care for you. Can you do that for me?" She looked at me and said, "Yes, I know, I know he is a great son! I will try." I gave her a hug and said, "that's all I can ask for. Thank you." I was grateful.

The support we hoped for from his sister is limited because she is busy volunteering at church and it's difficult for her to see her mother. So, much of the caregiving has fallen on Scott's shoulders and mine. Some of his sister's actions have caused him real pain; pain that does not disappear just because the day ends. So, when Scott comes home, exhausted and emotionally worn down, I am his safe place. And being his safe place means I often sense, his hurt, stress and pain.

Of course, I understand it, but understanding does not make it easy. That is why, one day, I called a friend. I did not call for advice. I did not call for solutions. I just needed to say out loud, "I am feeling a little stressed." My friend listened. And then said something simple but profoundly wise, "Everyone needs someone to vent to. And right now, your husband doesn't need you to fix anything. He just needs you to listen." That moment captured the heart of the Care Code.

Care is not always about doing. Support is not always about solving. Love is not always about saying the right thing. Sometimes, care is just presence. When someone needs to vent, your role is not to respond, not to analyze, not to correct, not to justify their feelings or tell them how to feel. You don't have to say anything at all. You just have to be there. Listen calmly, listen without interrupting, listen without judgment and listen without turning their pain into a project.

Consider this guiding mantra in your life, be there for someone who needs you and just let them VENT. That quiet, steady listening is not passive, it is powerful. It tells the other person, "You are safe here. Your feelings have somewhere to land."

My friend also shared something else that struck me deeply and aligns perfectly with the Care Code that we have been teaching our children, "Be careful who you choose to marry. Be careful who you choose as friends." Because when someone truly cares about you, their problems become your problems. And, when you truly care about them, your problems become theirs. That's not weakness, that is connection and that is the cycle of care.

The Care Code is not about having all the answers. It is about showing up with compassion, understanding that strength may mean silence and remembering that even caregivers need care. Sometimes the most loving thing you can offer another human being is not advice, but your quiet, unwavering presence.

Here is a Care Code principle, you do not have to fix someone's pain to care for them, sometimes the code is simply to listen.

So, be prepared to **Just Listen!**

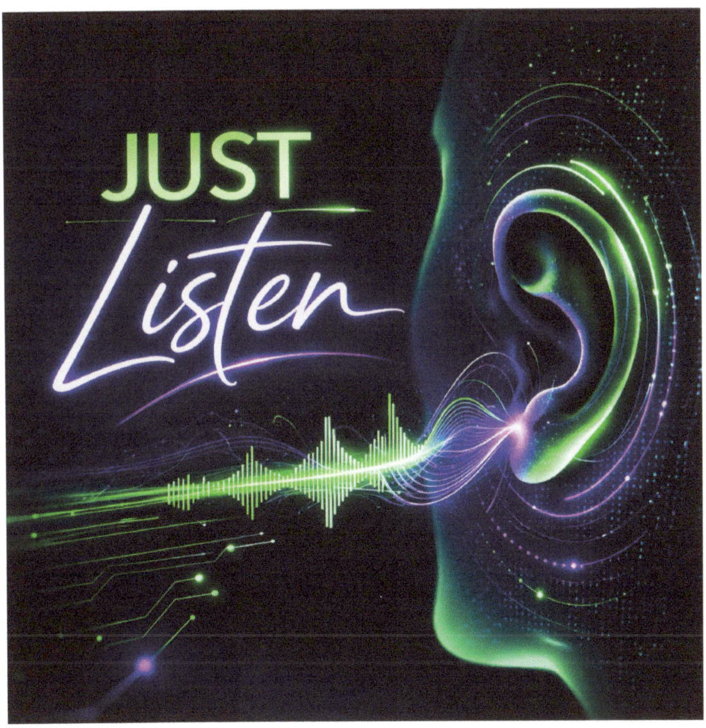

10

Get Off The Plane

There are moments in life when everything depends on one decision, one voice, one signal or one choice.

My husband was on a plane in Fort Lauderdale, headed to the Bahamas. He had been wearing his Rm2.ai™ device consistently, just as we encourage others to do. The purpose of the device is simple but powerful, monitor vitals continuously and reveal subtle changes that might otherwise go unnoticed.

The day before he boarded the plane, his heart rate had been erratic. It was not dramatic. It was not loud. It was not an emergency, yet. But, it was different. And different matters.

While on the plane waiting to take off, he began to feel unwell. The left side of his body tingled. Then it felt numb. A wave of discomfort and fear came upon him, subtle but undeniable. Many people would have dismissed it. Many would have waited. Many would have told themselves, I'll be fine. Instead, when the flight attendant asked him if he was alright, he said, "No, I need to get off this plane. I need to go to the emergency room." That decision may have saved his life.

911 was called. Paramedics came on the plane and transported him immediately to the nearest emergency room. His blood pressure on the ambulance was not extreme. Nothing appeared catastrophic. But something was not right.

As he was being transported to the emergency room, I checked his vitals remotely. Rm2.ai™ had captured and sent out two alerts the day before, showing an erratic heart rhythm. A pattern that did not belong. He shared that information with the doctors at the hospital. After numerous tests, five days in the hospital with two of them in the critical care unit, they confirmed it: he had experienced a mild stroke.

Strokes and heart attacks do not happen overnight. They build, they whisper and they shift subtly inside the body before they ever shout. What happened to my husband was not random. The signs were there. The body had been communicating. Rm2.ai™ early warning health intelligence had captured what the naked eye could not see.

He continued monitoring with Rm2.ai™ while in the hospital. The physician reviewed the trends. Upon discharge, the doctor advised him to continue monitoring with the Rm2.ai™ early warning health intelligence platform and to follow up with his doctor. The early warning mattered. It provided context. It gave insight. It told a story of what had been happening internally before the visible event occurred.

That is the essence of The Care Code. Crisis is rarely sudden. It is often unobserved or ignored. This chapter is not only about the Rm2.ai™ early warning health intelligence platform, it is also about humanity.

When he came home, weak and resting, relief flooded our home. But the next day, I found myself crying uncontrollably. I could not immediately explain why. Was it relief? Was it fear? Was it gratitude? It was exhausting. It was relief. Caring carries a heavy weight. When you are the caregiver, when you are the spouse, when you are the one watching vitals, answering calls, praying, hoping, bracing yourself for bad news, you carry a silent burden. And it is okay to feel it. It is okay to cry. It is okay to reach out.

During my husband's hospitalization, I felt the Care Code first hand. My family prayed. Our church members at St. Christophers prayed. My sorors prayed. Friends called. Messages poured in. The support reminded me of something profound, care is not weakness, care is strength. But strength requires support.

The Care Code is not only about protecting the ones we love. It is about protecting ourselves as caregivers. It is about recognizing that caring deeply does not mean carrying everything alone. It is about listening. Listening to the intelligence. Listening to the body. Listening to the quiet signals before they become alarms.

“Get off the plane” is more than a story. It is a principle. When your body signals that something is not right: get off the plane. When your vitals change: get off the plane. When something does not feel right: get off the plane. When intuition and information align: act. Do not wait for certainty. Do not wait for collapse or a crisis. Act early.

Prevention is the highest form of love. Monitoring what is happening inside gives us visibility before something irreversible happens. Rm2.ai™ helped reveal subtle changes in my husband’s heart rhythm before his stroke. We are grateful he was wearing it. We are grateful he spoke up. We are grateful he got off the plane.

Live on, live well, pay attention and appreciate every moment. And when your body speaks, listen. Because sometimes survival depends on one courageous decision. Get off the plane.

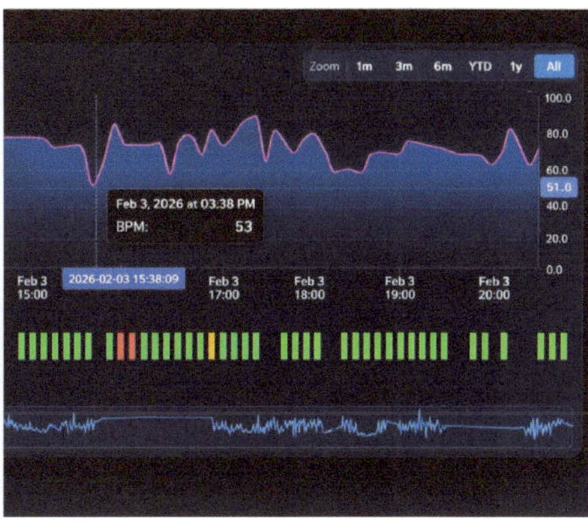

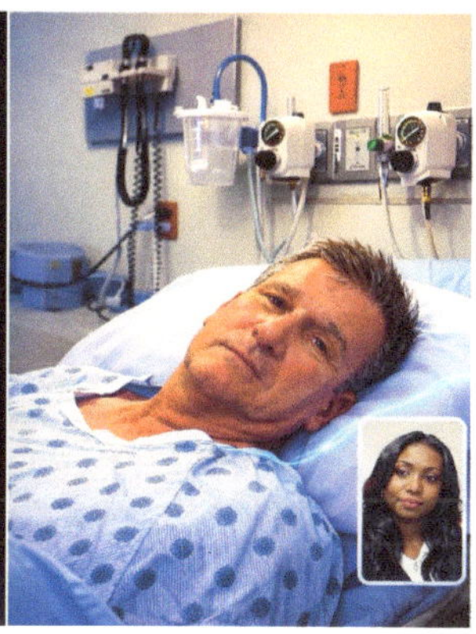

February 4, 2026

11

The Financial Burden of Reactive Care

The most expensive care is the care that came too late. Healthcare costs are rising at an unsustainable pace not because people are living longer, but because systems are reacting too late. Emergency room visits, hospital admissions, preventable complications and avoidable readmissions are driving billions of dollars in unnecessary spending each year.

The truth is simple and uncomfortable. Many high-cost healthcare events were preventable. Falls, dehydration, medication errors, missed early symptoms and cognitive decline go unnoticed until crisis. These are not sudden events, they are the result of missed signals, delayed responses and fragmented care. Prevention is no longer a "nice to have." It is the only viable path forward.

Traditional healthcare has long operated on a reactive model, waiting until illness or injury is advanced enough to require clinical intervention. This design fundamentally undermines patient outcomes, inflates costs and contributes to systemic dysfunction.

Reactive care delays intervention until harm has already occurred. Under this model, clinicians focus predominantly on treating symptoms and advanced disease rather than preventing illness and promoting wellness. The consequence is that patients often seek help only after their condition has progressed, leading to poorer health trajectories and a heavier clinical burden on providers (MDI Health Analytics, 2025).

It drives excessive healthcare spending with limited return. In 2024, in the U.S., an estimated 90 percent of the $5.3 trillion annual healthcare expenditure was directed toward managing chronic and mental health conditions. Many of which are preventable or could be mitigated through earlier, proactive care (MDI Health Analytics, 2025).

Patients who postpone care until symptoms escalate often experience complications that could have been prevented with earlier intervention. Evidence from chronic disease research demonstrates that delayed care correlates with significantly worse physical and mental health outcomes.

Provider burnout is both a symptom and amplifier of reactive systems. Healthcare workers in reactive environments face relentless pressures to respond to acute problems with insufficient time, support or resources. National surveys estimate that 35 – 50 percent of nurses and physicians report symptoms of burnout. These rates are well above many other professions. This burnout is associated with increased medical errors, communication failures and worse, patient safety outcomes (CDC, 2024).

The impact of burnout directly affects patient care quality. Burnout among clinical staff has been linked with adverse safety events, reduced team effectiveness and lower patient satisfaction, eroding trust in the system and compounding the very problems reactive care seeks to solve. (CDC, 2024).

Reactive care strains emergency services and inflates costs unnecessarily. Patients with conditions that could have been managed earlier often end up in emergency departments, driving up wait times and diverting resources from true emergencies. Proactive care strategies are associated with up to 30 percent lower overall healthcare costs by reducing preventable hospital admissions and intensive treatments (MyDecine, 2024).

Reactive care cost the system and patients. The United States spends an extraordinary amount on healthcare, yet most of that spending goes toward treating illness after harm has already occurred. The $5.3 trillion spending is a

7.2 percent increase from the previous year, representing nearly 18 percent of the nation's GDP (CMS, 2024). On a per-person basis, this amounts to about $15,474 annually. This staggering expenditure reflects a system designed around reactive care, intervening only after disease has already progressed.

By contrast, proactive care which emphasizes prevention, early detection and long-term health management has the potential to dramatically reduce both suffering and financial burden. Actuarial research from Deloitte projects that by 2040, a shift to proactive care could generate up to $2.2 trillion in annual U.S. system savings, primarily through reduced medical and prescription costs (Deloitte, 2025). Medicare alone could see savings exceeding $500 billion per year, while proactive management of chronic conditions such as diabetes, heart disease and cancer could cut more than $700 billion annually in healthcare expenditures. For individuals, this shift could reduce per-person healthcare costs by over $7,000 each year (Deloitte, 2025).

To put these figures in perspective, the current total U.S. healthcare spending of approximately $5.3 trillion could be offset by proactive strategies, reducing per-person costs from $15,474 to roughly $8,400. Medicare's annual spending of $848 billion could be trimmed by more than $500 billion, while chronic disease management alone offers potential annual savings exceeding $700 billion. Altogether, the system could save $2.2 trillion per year, transforming both public and private healthcare landscapes (CMS, 2024; Deloitte, 2025).

These numbers matter because reactive care waits until disease has struck, already incurring massive costs. Proactive care intercepts risk early, reducing the intensity of treatment, preventing hospitalizations and mitigating long-term complications. For families, this means thousands of dollars in individual savings and for society, it translates to trillions in system-wide efficiency gains. These statistics are a mandate, healthcare should be designed around preserving health before a crisis, not reacting after it.

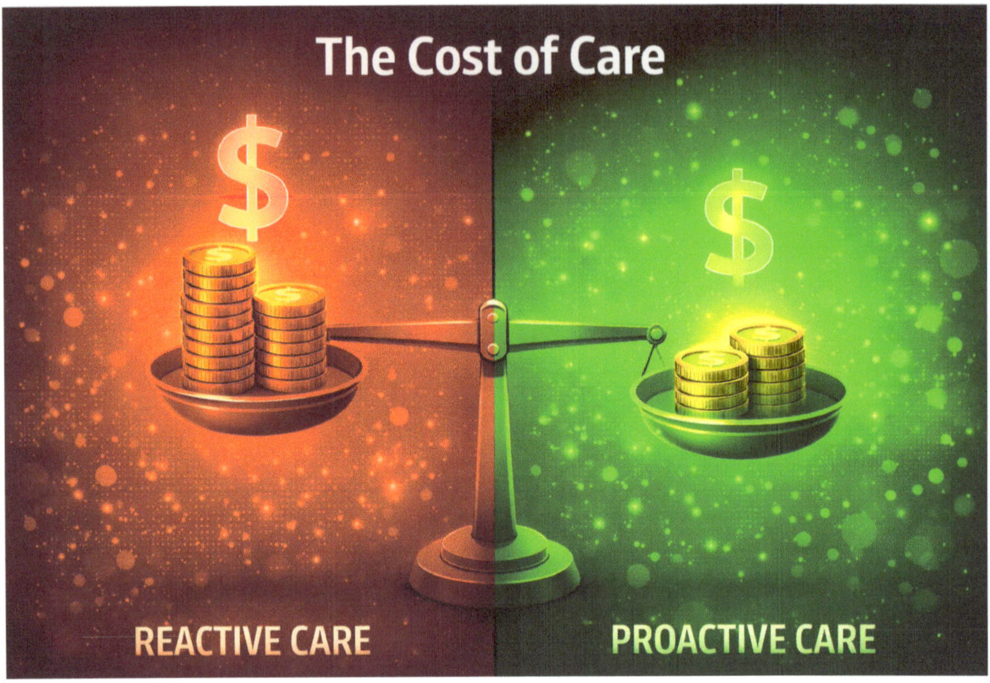
The Cost of Care
REACTIVE CARE
PROACTIVE CARE

12

Reducing Healthcare Costs Through Prevention

Prevention changes the cost curve. Preventive care is often misunderstood as simply more doctor visits or additional tests, but it is far more strategic than that. It is about earlier awareness, smarter monitoring and timely action. This is exactly where early warning health intelligence transforms the healthcare equation. When risks are identified early, small issues stay small, interventions are simpler and less expensive, seniors remain independent longer, families experience fewer crises and healthcare systems avoid unnecessary utilization.

Early warning health intelligence enables cost-saving prevention. Rm2.ai™ LiveVital Intelligence is a continuous monitoring tool, designed to be a preventive intelligence system. It continuously scans for patterns that humans may miss, including subtle changes in vitals, mobility that increase fall risk, missed medications that lead to complications, shifts in sleep, activity, or social interaction. Instead of reacting to emergencies, Rm2.ai™ early warning health intelligence platform is designed to identify health trends early, alert families and care teams. This enables timely, low-cost interventions, and prevents escalation into high-cost events.

The financial impact of prevention indicates that every prevented fall can save thousands of dollars, every avoided hospitalization can save tens of thousands and every delayed nursing home placement preserves both independence and dignity. On a broader scale, proactive interventions contribute to systemic savings. Considering that reactive care costs the U.S. healthcare system $5.3

trillion annually (CMS, 2024), proactive strategies that reduce hospitalizations, readmissions and long-term care utilization can shift the financial trajectory by trillions. Actuarial projections suggest that proactive care could save up to $2.2 trillion per year, with Medicare alone saving $500 billion and chronic disease prevention accounting for $700 billion in annual savings (Deloitte, 2025). On an individual level, per-person healthcare costs could be reduced by over $7,000 annually.

For patients, this translates into fewer emergency visits, fewer hospital stays, better quality of life and extended independence. Families benefit from reduced out-of-pocket costs, fewer missed workdays and lower emotional and financial stress. Providers see improved outcomes, reduced readmissions and enhanced care coordination. For healthcare systems and governments, preventive technology supports lower hospitalization rates, reduced long-term care costs, improved population health metrics and more sustainable spending.

Prevention is not just compassion, but is economically responsible as well. Rm2.ai™ early warning health intelligence platform turns prevention into a measurable, scalable strategy, transforming healthcare from a reactive cost center into a value-based system where early interventions save money, preserve dignity and improve lives.

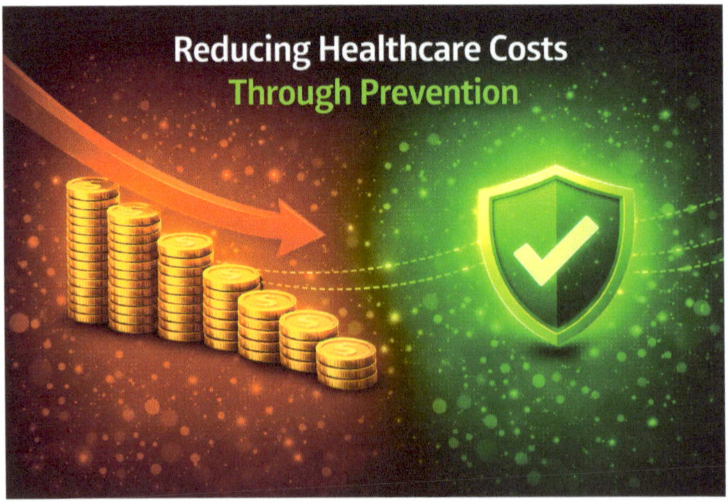

13

The Invisible Killer: What's Inside Matters Most

In 2024, my cousin died of a massive heart attack. He was 58 years old. He looked fine, no warning, no collapse in public, no obvious sign that his life was moments away from ending. He woke up, waited for his wife to walk their daughter to the bus, and then, he was gone.

What haunts those left behind is not just the loss. It's the question that never stops echoing: How did we not know? Could we have done something to help? The truth is devastating and simple. No one was monitoring what was happening inside his body. His vitals were silent. His heart was struggling quietly. And the outside gave no clues. This is one of the most dangerous myths in caregiving and health: If someone looks okay, they must be okay.

The Care Code exists to dismantle that lie because what's happening inside the body matters far more than what we can see with our eyes. Blood pressure rises long before collapse, heart rhythms change before chest pain appears, oxygen drops before breathing looks labored and stress silently taxes the heart before anyone says, "I don't feel well." The body whispers long before it screams and when no one is listening people die.

My cousin didn't fail to care for himself. His family didn't fail him, the system failed to monitor what mattered. We live in a world where we monitor packages, bank accounts and smartphones in real time but not the human heart beating inside the people we love most. That is not a technology gap, it is a care gap. Rm2.ai™ early warning health intelligence platform was built to close that gap. It does not rely on appearances, it does not wait for symptoms, it does not assume "fine" means okay or safe.

Rm2.ai™ early warning health intelligence platform monitors what's happening on the inside, heart rate, vital signs, pattern changes that the human eye can't detect. It is designed to predict health trends early. It turns invisible danger into visible data and data into action. Rm2.ai™ care is sent in the form of automatic alerts. This is not about fear, it's about love expressed as vigilance.

Because love is not simply showing up when something goes wrong, love is preventing the moment that changes everything. If someone had been monitoring my cousin's vitals, if changes had been detected, if an alert had been raised before his heart gave out, if, if. There is no guarantee. But there was a chance and chances matter!

The Care Code is not about replacing human connection, it is about protecting it. It is about saying, "I love you enough to watch over what you cannot feel, see, or articulate."

Inside monitoring is not intrusive, it is protective, it is compassionate, it is responsible. We cannot keep relying on "he looked fine" as a care strategy because the outside lies, but the inside tells the truth. Rm2.ai™ listens to that truth quietly, constantly and without judgment so families do not have to live with the words, "If only we had known."

The Care Code exists for every spouse, child, friend, and family member who has lost someone suddenly. For everyone who has said, "There were no signs." For everyone who wishes love had come with an early warning health intelligence platform, this is for you. Care is not passive, care is proactive, care monitors what others can not see. That is how love shows up, before it is too late. That is The Care Code!

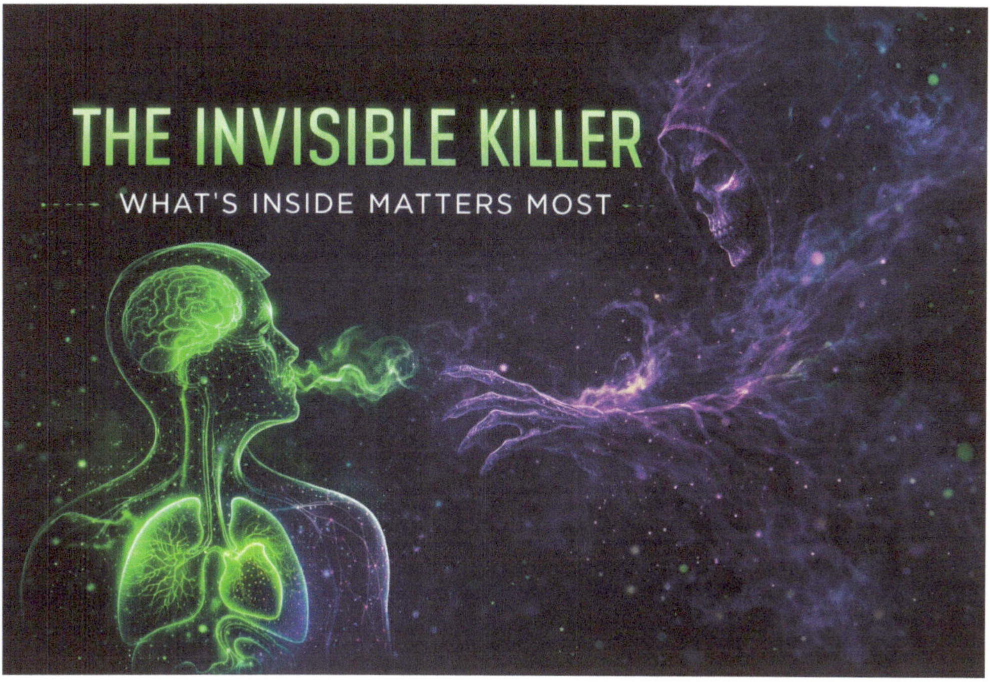
THE INVISIBLE KILLER
WHAT'S INSIDE MATTERS MOST

14

The True Cost of Doing Nothing

The economic and emotional price of broken care is substantial. The true cost of broken care is far greater than what typical healthcare accounting captures. Traditional healthcare systems measure cost per admission, cost per bed per day and readmission expenses. However, they rarely account for the financial and emotional toll borne by families and caregivers. In the United States alone, family caregivers provide an estimated 36 billion hours of unpaid care valued at roughly $600 billion annually, equivalent to the GDP of major industries and representing work that would otherwise require a paid workforce (NCCDP, 2025).

This unpaid labor masks a deeper economic strain. Nearly 56 percent of working caregivers report work-related strain, including reduced hours or taking time off. Additionally, about 18 percent reduce work hours while 9 percent leave the workforce entirely, leading to lost wages, benefits and future retirement savings (NCCDP, 2025).

Caregivers often spend around 20 percent of their income on caregiving-related expenses, dipping into savings, cutting essentials and delaying their own healthcare to make ends meet (United For ALICE, 2024).

The cost is beyond dollars. There are costs that no ledger shows: the panic of missed warning signs or the sleepless nights. Also, the anxiety after emergency hospitalizations, the emotional exhaustion of balancing caregiving with life's other demands and the guilt that follows preventable crises. For seniors themselves, a fall, dehydration crisis, or hospital admission often triggers a loss of confidence, fear of living alone, accelerated functional decline and a diminished sense of autonomy costs that ripple through every aspect of life.

Preliminary data from remote monitoring and predictive care research suggest these problems can be mitigated. Studies on remote patient monitoring suggest reductions in hospital readmissions by 15–45 percent and annual per patient savings of $1,200–$4,000 or more by preventing complications and lowering hospitalization costs (Remington Report, 2024).

Machine learning models show that high medication adherence and preventive care can reduce hospitalization risk by more than 37 percent, illustrating the power of predictive, data-driven intervention (Zhang & Chen, 2025).

Doing nothing, however, is not neutral. It is the most expensive decision of all. When crises occur, families shoulder hidden costs. Lost income from caregivers leaving jobs, emergency room bills that skyrocket without warning, long-term anxiety that affects productivity and the emotional trauma of watching someone they love suffer preventable decline. What healthcare systems label "unavoidable" is often predictable and avoidable with foresight and early action.

The emotional economics of care are real. Burnout among caregivers leads to poorer health, higher rates of missed appointments and medication errors. Ultimately lending to more expensive crisis-driven care. When families are empowered with real-time data and early warnings, they intervene earlier, communicate with clinicians more effectively and avoid crisis-driven decisions that impact lives and finances alike.

Prevention is not a cost center, it is an emotional and economic investment. When families trust the system and stay engaged, when they receive clear, actionable insights, they make better decisions to avoid crises, protect independence and preserve dignity. The question is no longer, "Can we afford prevention?" The real question is "Can we afford the cost of doing nothing?"

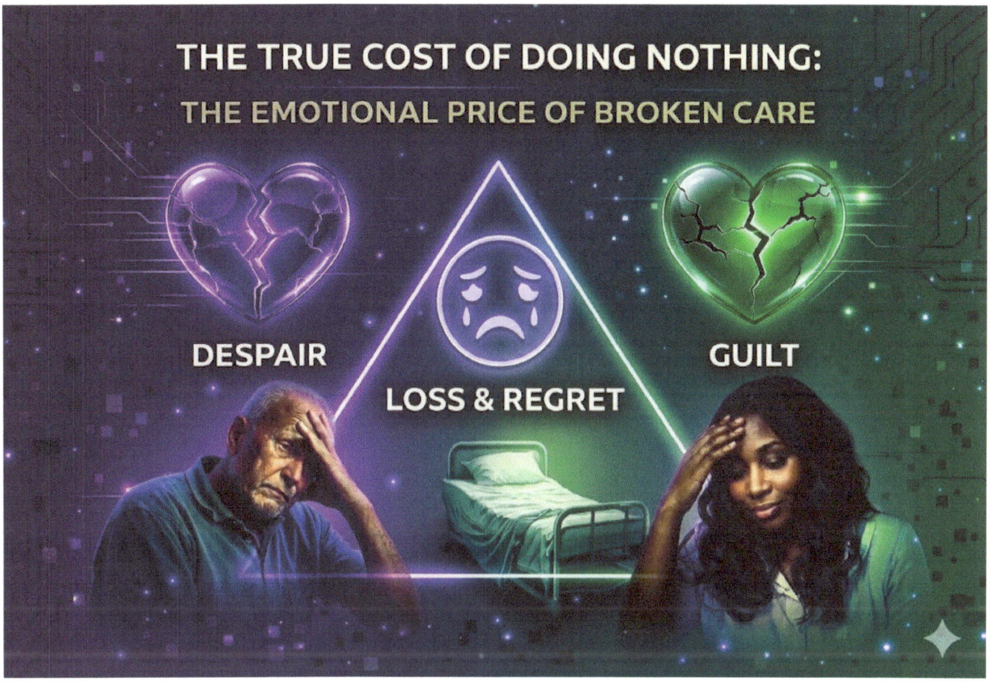

15

The Uncomfortable Truth: Caring During The Final Stages

There is a part of caregiving we rarely talk about not because it is not important, but because it is uncomfortable: dying. On January 23, 2026, that discomfort became impossible to ignore.

My husband's blood pressure spiked to 200/115. He was visibly shaken, overwhelmed and terrified not just for himself, but for his mother. She is in an assisted living facility and is afraid. She needs our support and love.

She calls him every 20 to 30 minutes. Sometimes 15 times a day. Each call carries fear, loneliness and a plea from her no one wants to say out loud: "Please don't leave me alone."

Every call elevated his stress and every unanswered ring carried guilt. Now slowly and silently, the caregiver was becoming the next patient. As his wife, I knew we had crossed a line from caring for someone to losing ourselves in care. So, we called our family physician, Dr. Michelle C. Powell. What she said changed everything.

She acknowledged the truth most families struggle to say or admit. His mother may be dying. She is afraid and wants someone with her every moment. But then Dr. Powell said something profound and freeing: "She may be dying, but her son still has to live." Wow! That sentence reframed everything.

Dr. Powell reminded us that love does not mean unlimited sacrifice. That caregiving without boundaries becomes dangerous. That guilt driven care can make the living sick. Her guidance was clear and compassionate. She increased my husband's blood pressure medication, advised him to get fresh air and walk to reset his nervous system. She caringly advised us to set boundaries and most importantly use tools to reduce constant emotional crisis.

This is where The Care Code becomes real. We implemented structure instead of panic and support instead of constant reaction. A camera was placed in his mother's room, so when she called, he could see she was safe. She began wearing her Rm2.ai™ early warning health intelligence device so he could monitor her vitals without rushing into fear. Now, he could check her vitals, movement and safety remotely. He could call her through the device, reassure her and respond with intention instead of urgency.

The result wasn't less love, it was better love. This early warning intelligence technology did not replace compassion, it protected it. This is the uncomfortable truth about dying and caregiving. Fear increases at the end of life, calls increase, needs escalate and without support: caregivers break.

The Care Code is not about avoiding death, it is about navigating it with clarity, dignity and boundaries. It teaches us that supporting someone does not mean abandoning yourself. Monitoring is not neglect, it is protection. Boundaries are not cruelty: they are important for survival.

This chapter exists because families everywhere are living this moment right now like us, silently, feeling guilty and utterly exhausted.

The Care Code gives language to the unspoken, tools for the unbearable and permission to care without collapsing. Remember caring at the end of life should never mean losing the lives of those still living. That is the Care Code.

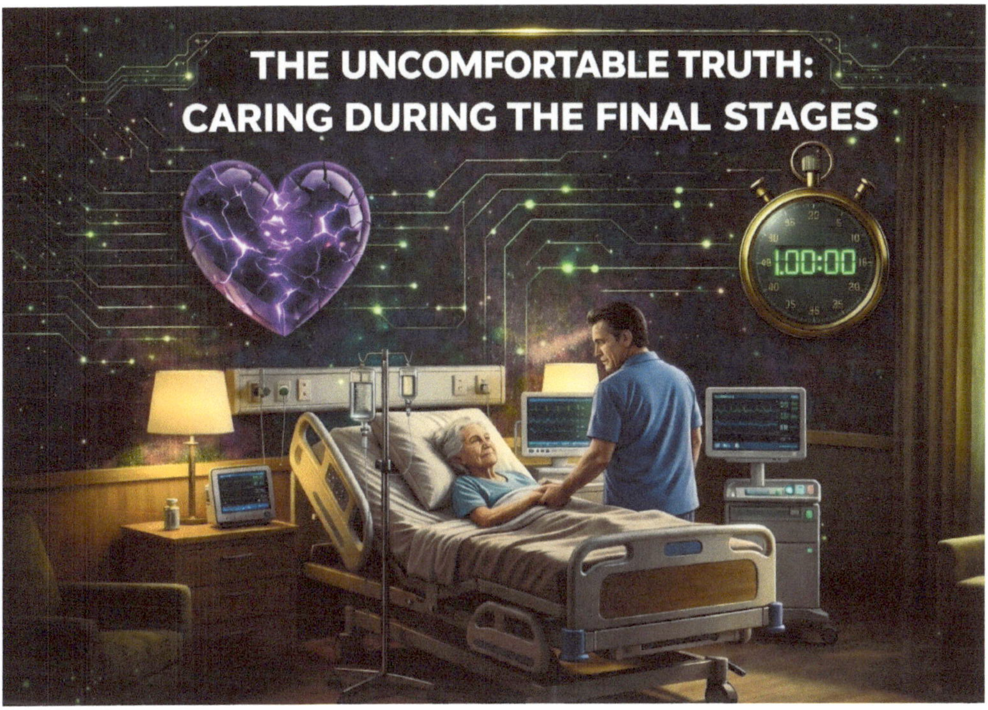
THE UNCOMFORTABLE TRUTH:
CARING DURING THE FINAL STAGES
1:00:00

16

The Care Code Manifesto

A call for a smarter, more human future is not the end, it is the beginning. Every generation is remembered for the problems it chooses to solve. We are living longer than ever before but we are not living better.

We have more data than any generation in history, yet we still react too late. We have the technology to prevent suffering, yet we wait for a crisis. The Care Code exists because waiting is no longer acceptable.

The Care Code is more than ideas. It is about responsibility. The truth is we can no longer ignore what is right in front of us. Healthcare today is built to respond, not to protect. It pays extensively for emergencies, not early warnings. It reacts to decline instead of preserving dignity. Most hospitalizations are preventable, most crises send signals in advance and most families would act, if they only knew sooner. Failure is not a lack of care, it is a lack of insight. Caring is taking action and doing to prevent versus react.

The Care Code Manifesto is a simple belief that prevention is the highest form of care. Early warnings save lives, protect dignity and reduce unnecessary and astronomical health care costs. Technology should serve humanity, not replace it. It must provide families clarity instead of chaos and support caregivers so they can avoid burnout. Seniors deserve independence and visibility, not isolation. Healthcare must be proactive, predictive and personal. This is the Care Code. A commitment to caring that empowers, protects and transforms the way we support those we love.

Rm2.ai™ changes everything. It is not a device. It is not an app. It is not a dashboard. It is an early warning health intelligence platform designed to predict health trends early, prevent avoidable hospital visits and protect dignity and independence ultimately impacting life and health span. By continuously monitoring vitals, falls, hydration, movement, trends and location, Rm2.ai™ transforms silence into signals, data into decisions, fear into foresight and crisis into prevention. It is designed to provide proactive support to families, caregivers and systems to send automatic alerts early. This is not futuristic. This is now.

We have a choice before us. Each reader of this book now faces a choice to continue reacting or start preventing, accept crisis as "normal" or demand better, treat aging as decline or protect longevity. The Care Code is not optional.

You have a role in the movement. This movement needs families who demand early warnings, caregivers who embrace smarter tools, healthcare leaders who redesign care models, policymakers who fund prevention and innovators who put humanity first to act. When we predict early, when we prevent harm, when we protect dignity, when we preserve health span and when we take action, we unlock The Care Code.

Will you be the one to take action? You are not just a reader. You are now a Code Breaker.

The Care Code Commitment

I commit to caring early and being attentive before challenges arise. I will remain mindful of the signals that health, safety and well-being may need attention. I embrace the belief that prevention is the highest form of care. I will strive to honor dignity, independence and quality of life for those I love.

Name: ________________________ Sign: ________________________

Date: ____________________

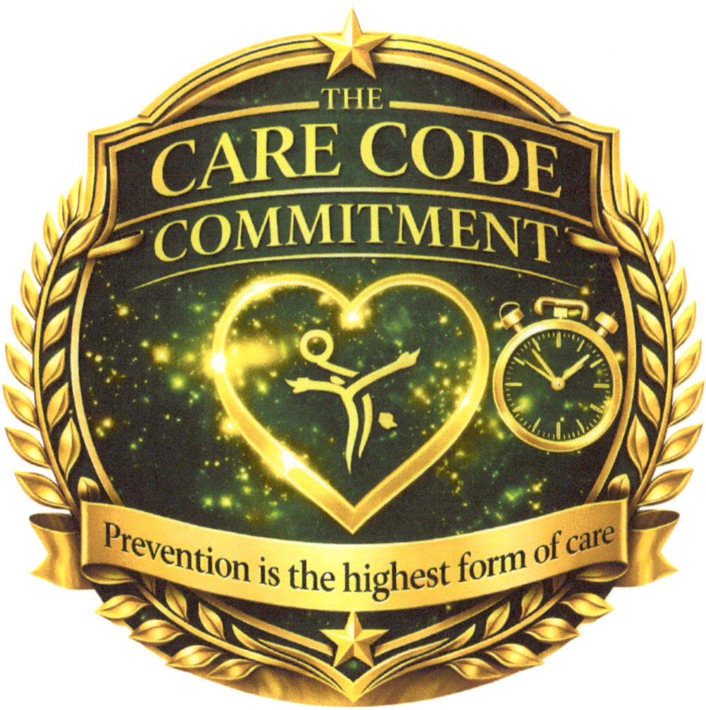

17

Conclusion

Care does not fail all at once. It fails quietly. It's missed signals, delayed action, assumptions that "this is just aging" and systems designed to respond after harm has already occurred.

The Care Code was written to interrupt that pattern. Throughout The Care Code, we have seen a simple yet powerful truth emerge again and again. Most crises do not arrive without warning. Falls, dehydration, medication errors, cognitive decline, caregiver burnout: these are rarely sudden. They are preceded by signals we overlook, patterns we dismiss and systems that wait too long to act.

But it does not have to be this way. We are living in a moment of extraordinary possibility. For the first time, we have the tools to predict risk early, prevent harm before it escalates and protect dignity while preserving independence. Technology when used thoughtfully and compassionately gives us the chance to move care upstream, where it belongs.

Tools alone are not enough. The Care Code is not just about AI, wearables or data. It is about intentional action. It is about families choosing to pay attention sooner. Caregivers being supported instead of stretched to the breaking point. Health systems shifting from reaction to prevention. And leaders having the courage to redesign care around people, not profit, convenience or outdated models.

Empowerment begins with awareness. Hope begins with action. If you are a family member, your next step is to stop waiting for a crisis to justify concern. Trust what you notice. Ask better questions. Advocate earlier. Caring smarter is not abandoning love, it is strengthening it.

If you are a caregiver, know this, burnout is not a personal failure. It is a system failure. You deserve support, insight and tools that help you care without sacrificing yourself.

If you are a healthcare leader, policymaker or innovator, the message is clear: the cost of doing nothing is no longer acceptable. Preventable harm is expensive in dollars, dignity, and lives. The future of care demands systems that are proactive, predictive and personal.

And if you are aging yourself as we all are, The Care Code is a reminder that independence is not lost overnight. It is preserved through awareness, early intervention and a commitment to care that sees you before you fall.

Cracking the Care Code is not about perfection. It is about paying attention sooner, acting with intention and choosing dignity every time. The future of care is not something we are waiting for. It is something we are building right now. Because care is not reactive, it is intentional.

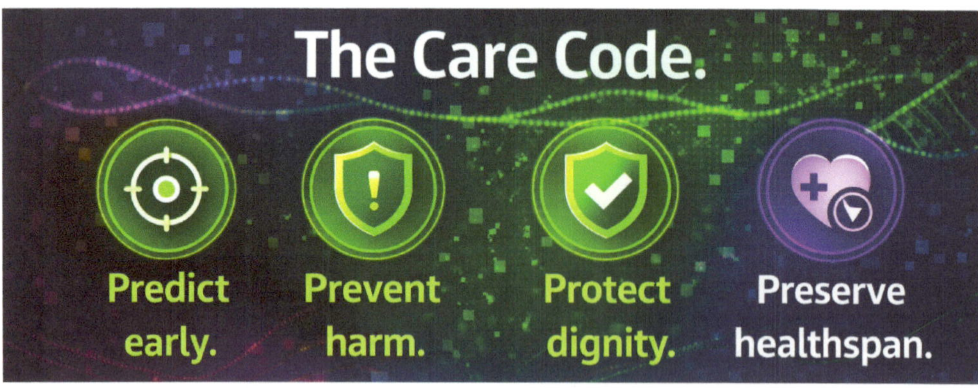
The Care Code.
Predict early.
Prevent harm.
Protect dignity.
Preserve healthspan.

Are You Missing the Signals? Self-Assessment

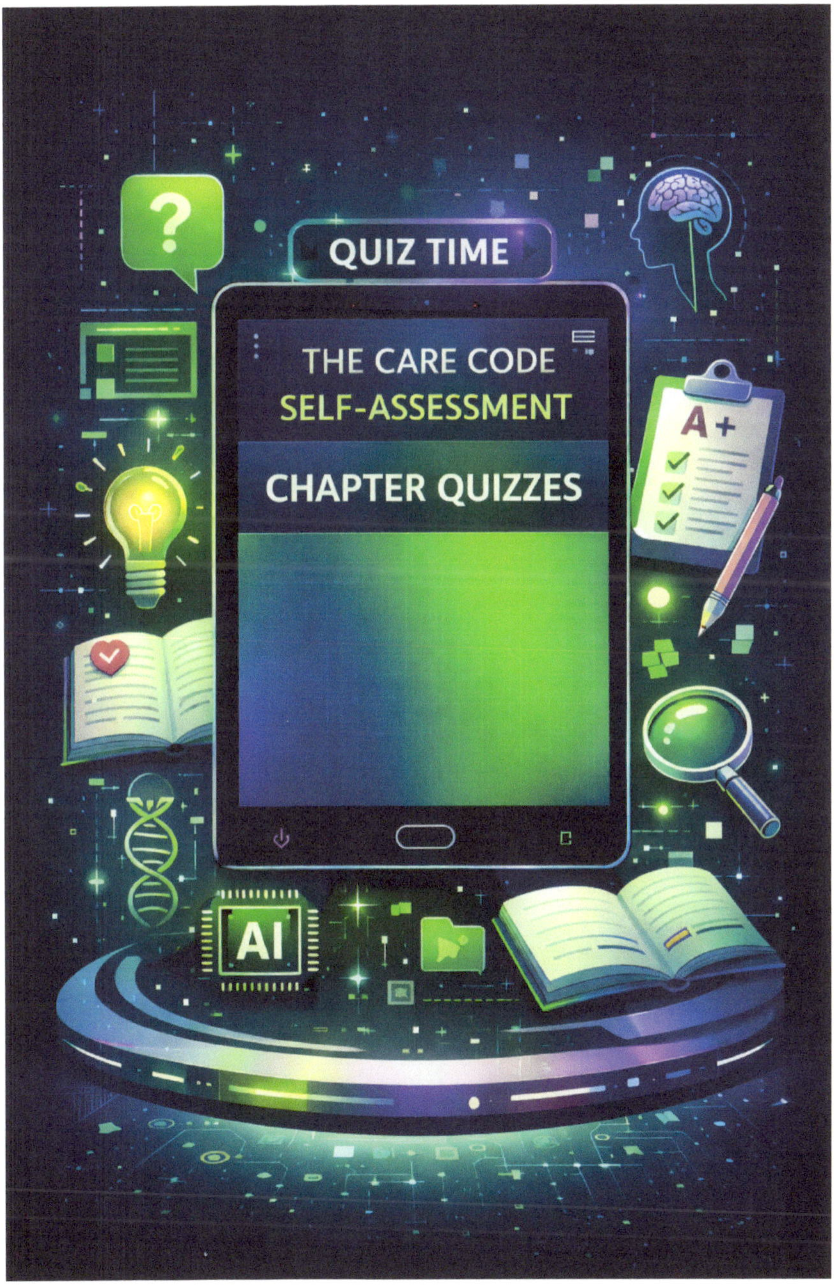

1

Why Health Care Needs Innovation

PURPOSE: To show how early warning + innovation leads to better outcomes versus waiting for a crisis.

THE SCENARIO: A senior living at home starts sleeping more, missing medications occasionally and moving less. Nothing seems urgent yet.

THE QUESTION: What is the BEST response?

CHOOSE ONE ACTION

A. Do nothing and assume it's normal aging.

B. Wait until a medical emergency happens.

C. Use AI and monitoring tools to detect trends and intervene early.

C. Use AI and monitoring tools to detect trends and intervene early

READER WORKSHEET

1. Today's healthcare system is mostly:

____

2. Early warning signs are important because they:

____

3. AI helps healthcare by:

____

✓ Identifying patterns
✓ Sending early alerts
✓ Supporting caregivers
✓ Preventing crises

4. Complete the sentence:
Innovation in healthcare means moving from reaction to

____.

5. True or False:
Waiting until symptoms are severe leads to better outcomes.

____

You've unlocked the FIRST Care Code.

1.Reactive. 2. Appear before emergencies and allow prevention 3. All of the above. 4.
Reaction → Prevention 5. False

2

The AI Advantage

PURPOSE: To show how AI turns information into early insight, giving caregivers and families an advantage they have never had before.

THE SCENARIO: A senior's vitals, activity, sleep, and hydration are being monitored. Each change alone seems minor but together they tell a story.

THE QUESTION: What gives AI the advantage over traditional care?

CHOOSE ONE ACTION

A. AI replaces doctors and caregivers.

B. AI analyzes patterns over time and alerts humans early.

C. AI only matters during emergencies.

B. AI analyzes patterns over time and alerts humans early

READER WORKSHEET

1. The main advantage of AI in healthcare is:

2. AI is most valuable when it is used to:

3. True or False:
AI replaces human caregivers.

4. AI helps caregivers by:

✔ Monitoring trends
✔ Sending alerts
✔ Supporting better decisions
✔ Reducing guesswork

5. Complete the sentence:
The AI advantage in healthcare is:

You've unlocked the AI Advantage and another Care Code.

1.Detecting patterns and risks early. 2. Prevent problems before they become emergencies. 3. False. 4. All of the above. 5. Early insight that enables prevention

4

The Predictive Power of Data

PURPOSE: To show how data trends allow caregivers and healthcare systems to predict problems before they happen, not react after damage is done.

THE SCENARIO: Over several weeks, a senior's data shows slight changes, lower activity, rising heart rate, poor sleep and missed hydration goals. No single reading is alarming but the pattern is.

THE QUESTION: What makes data predictive rather than just informative?

CHOOSE ONE ACTION

A. Looking at one data point at a time.
B. Waiting until values reach emergency levels.
C. Analyzing trends and patterns over time.

C. Analyzing trends and patterns over time

READER WORKSHEET

1. Predictive data focuses on:

____

2. Why are trends more valuable than single readings?

____

3. True or False:
Waiting for emergency thresholds leads to better outcomes.

____

4. Predictive data helps prevent:
✔ Falls
✔ Hospitalizations
✔ Medical crises
✔ Rapid decline

5. Complete the sentence:
Predictive data allows caregivers to act:

____

You've unlocked the Predictive Power of Data and another Care Code.

1.Trends over time. 2. They reveal early risk before a crisis occurs. 3. False. 4. All of the above. 5. Before a crisis occurs.

5

Early Warnings Save Lives

PURPOSE: To demonstrate how responding to early warning signs may prevent crises and save lives.

THE SCENARIO: A senior shows several subtle changes over two weeks: reduced appetite, missed medications, lower activity, and disrupted sleep. No emergency has occurred.

THE QUESTION: What is the BEST response?

CHOOSE ONE ACTION

A. Wait until symptoms become severe.

B. Address each issue only if it becomes urgent.

C. Respond early using monitoring, data, and caregiver support.

C. Respond early using monitoring, data, and caregiver support.

READER WORKSHEET

1. Early warning signs are:

____

2. Why are early warnings so powerful?

____

3. True or False:
Most medical crises happen without warning.

____

4. Early warnings help prevent:

____

✔ Falls
✔ Hospitalizations
✔ Rapid decline
✔ Loss of independence

5. Complete the sentence:
Early warnings save lives by allowing care to begin

____

You've unlocked another Care Code and learned the importance of early warnings.

1.Subtle changes that appear before a crisis. 2. They allow intervention before crisis occurs. 3. False. 4. All of the above. 5. Before a crisis occurs.

6

Empowering Families and Caregivers

PURPOSE: To show how access to information and early alerts empowers caregivers to provide better, calmer, and more effective care.

THE SCENARIO: A caregiver lives in another city and worries constantly about their loved one's safety, health and daily routines. Updates only come after something goes wrong.

THE QUESTION: What empowers caregivers the most?

CHOOSE ONE ACTION

A. Relying on emergency calls and hospital updates.
B. Constantly checking in and hoping for the best.
C. Having real-time data, alerts, and early warning insights.

C. Having real-time data, alerts, and early warning insights

READER WORKSHEET

1. Caregiver empowerment means:

____

2. What causes caregiver burnout?

____

3. True or False:
Empowering caregivers removes the human element of care.

____

4. Empowered caregivers are better able to:

____

- ✔ Make informed decisions
- ✔ Communicate with providers
- ✔ Prevent crises
- ✔ Maintain their own well-being

5. Complete the sentence:
Empowering caregivers leads to__________________________ care for seniors.

You've unlocked another Care Code and strengthened the circle of care.

1.Having information, tools, and support to act early. 2. Lack of visibility, constant worry, and reactive care. 3. False. 4. All of the above. 5. Safer, calmer, and more consistent.

8

Dignity, Independence and Aging in Place

PURPOSE: To show how early support and intelligent monitoring preserve dignity and independence.

THE SCENARIO: A senior wants to remain at home. Family members worry about safety and are considering moving them into an assisted living despite no major incident yet.

THE QUESTION: What is the BEST approach?

CHOOSE ONE ACTION

A. Move the senior immediately to ensure safety.
B. Limit independence to reduce risk.
C. Use early warning tools to support safe aging in place.

C. Use early warning tools to support safe aging in place

READER WORKSHEET

1. Aging in place means:

____

2. What most threatens senior independence?

____

3. True or False:
Safety requires giving up dignity.

____

4. Early warning tools help seniors:

✔ Stay in their homes longer
✔ Avoid unnecessary moves
✔ Maintain autonomy
✔ Feel secure

5. Complete the sentence:
Dignity in care is preserved when support is

____

You've unlocked another Care Code and protected independence.

1. Living safely at home with the right support. 2. Lack of visibility and early warning. 3. False. 4. All of the above. 5. Respectful, timely, and unobtrusive.

One PROMISE TO YOURSELF

Remember2™ Care for yourself because it protects the people you love. This is part of The Care Code.

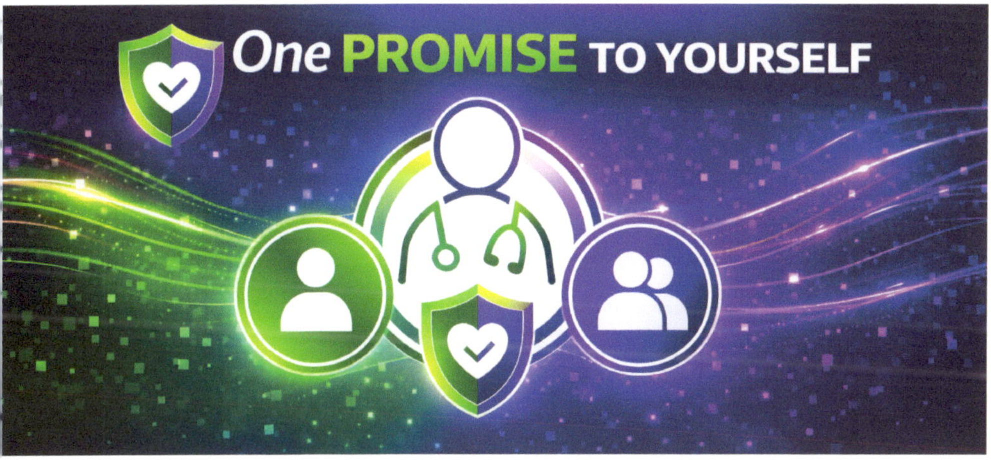

Appendix

The Care Code Practical Toolkit
Early Warning Sign Checklist

Use this checklist weekly to check on you and your loved one's well being. Small changes matter.

Physical Changes

□ Increased fatigue or weakness
□ Unsteady walking or new balance issues
□ Changes in appetite
□ Unexplained weight loss or gain
□ Shortness of breath
□ Swelling in legs or feet
□ Changes in sleep patterns
□ Frequent bathroom accidents

Cognitive Changes

□ Increased forgetfulness
□ Confusion about time or place
□ Difficulty following conversations
□ Repeating questions
□ Poor judgment

Emotional or Behavioral Changes

□ Withdrawal from activities
□ Irritability or mood swings
□ Anxiety or restlessness
□ Sudden apathy
□ Increased agitation

If two or more changes appear/occur within a short period, investigate early & consider contacting your medical provider.

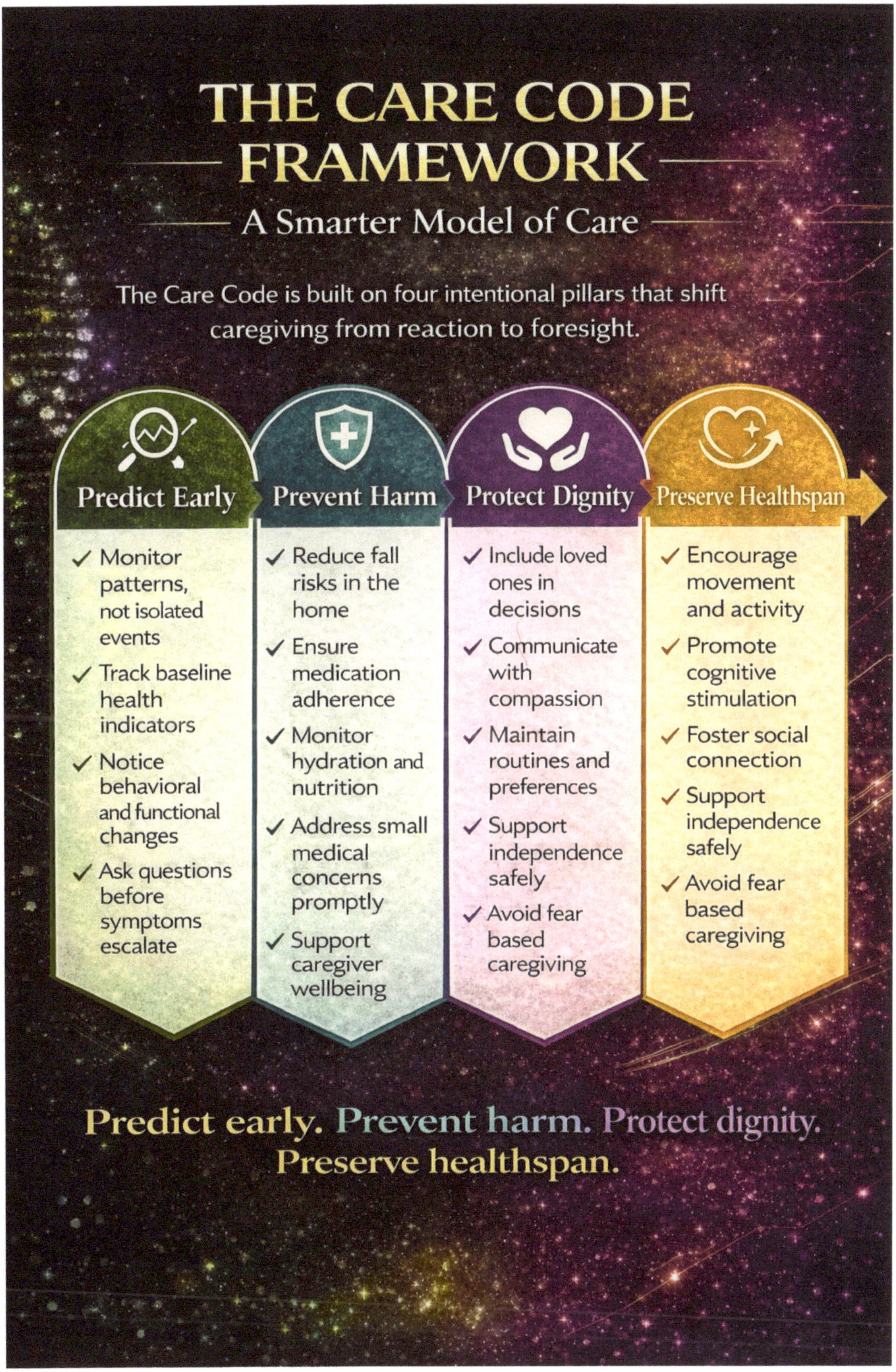
THE CARE CODE FRAMEWORK
A Smarter Model of Care
The Care Code is built on four intentional pillars that shift caregiving from reaction to foresight.
Predict Early
✓ Monitor patterns, not isolated events
✓ Track baseline health indicators
✓ Notice behavioral and functional changes
✓ Ask questions before symptoms escalate
Prevent Harm
✓ Reduce fall risks in the home
✓ Ensure medication adherence
✓ Monitor hydration and nutrition
✓ Address small medical concerns promptly
✓ Support caregiver wellbeing
Protect Dignity
✓ Include loved ones in decisions
✓ Communicate with compassion
✓ Maintain routines and preferences
✓ Support independence safely
✓ Avoid fear based caregiving
Preserve Healthspan
✓ Encourage movement and activity
✓ Promote cognitive stimulation
✓ Foster social connection
✓ Support independence safely
✓ Avoid fear based caregiving
Predict early. Prevent harm. Protect dignity. Preserve healthspan.

Acknowledgements

The Care Code exists because of the people who believed, supported, challenged and carried me along the way.

First and foremost, I thank my husband, Scott Johnson. Thank you for always believing in me, standing beside me through every season and supporting me without hesitation. You are an extraordinary husband, an incredible son and a devoted father. Your strength, compassion and commitment to family embody the very essence of The Care Code.

I also want to acknowledge my mother-in-law, Kathryn Johnson. Since her fall and hip fracture over a year and a half ago, she has been on a difficult, painful and demanding journey. I honor her strength, resilience and continued fight through difficult circumstances. I thank her for allowing us to show up, to care deeply and to live out The Care Code in real time. Her journey has taught us patience, compassion and what it truly means to stand by someone through adversity.

To Burton Firtel, founder of Remember2, Inc, thank you for your confidence in me and your belief in our shared vision. Your trust opened the door to an extraordinary journey, allowing us to develop a revolutionary ground breaking technology that truly serves others and provides proactive and preventative care.

To my Chief Operating Officer and dear friend, Vern Cameron, your unwavering support, wisdom, insight and friendship have been invaluable. I am deeply grateful for your leadership, perspective and steadfast belief in both the mission and in me.

To my dearest friend, Dr. Michelle C. Powell, I love you dearly. You have shown up for me and my family time and time again, without hesitation, at any hour. Your kindness, beauty and unwavering care exemplify The Care Code in its purest form. I am incredibly proud of you and of the way you carry your love for people into your service as a Physician and Councilwoman of Miami Gardens.

To my biological children, Angelo and Alexis, you are my heart. Your kindness, empathy, and support remind me daily why this work matters. You live The Care Code naturally and I am endlessly proud of the adults you are becoming. To my bonus children, Alexandra and Zachary, you have brought joy, laughter and love into my life in ways I never expected. Your kindness, openness, and support remind me that family is more than blood, it's heart and connection. Thank you for being a part of this journey and for allowing me to love you as my own.

To my friends, far too many to name, my sorors and church family, thank you for your encouragement, patience, prayers and love throughout this journey. Your support has meant more than you know.

To my sisters, Krista and Vonette, you are my backbone. Your strength, loyalty and constant presence have carried me more times than I can count. Thank you for always showing up to support me.

To my mother, Eunice Deveaux, thank you for shaping me into the woman I am today. You instilled in me a heart for service, love and leadership and taught me what it means to care deeply and lead with purpose.

Above all, I give thanks to my Lord and Savior, Jesus Christ. Thank you for the strength, courage and grace to live intentionally, love boldly and remain grounded in faith. Even in moments of doubt, criticism and misunderstanding, You gave me the resolve to choose kindness, remain true to myself and walk daily in the principles of The Care Code.

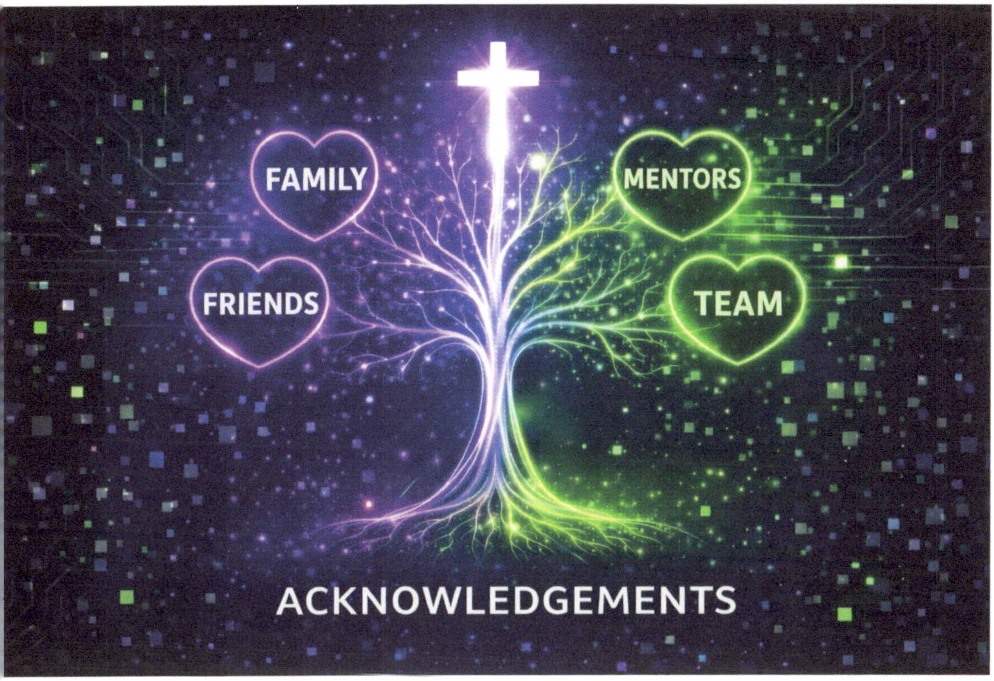
FAMILY
MENTORS
FRIENDS
TEAM
ACKNOWLEDGEMENTS

About the Author

Corlette Deveaux is an entrepreneur, author, inventor and senior care innovator dedicated to transforming how aging adults and individuals with chronic conditions are supported. She is the CEO and Co-Founder of Remember2 Inc. an AI-powered early warning health intelligence platform created to shift healthcare from reactive response to proactive, predictive and dignity-centered care.

A former owner of A Joyful Heart Adult Day Care, Corlette brings rare firsthand experience from the front lines of caregiving. Her work is shaped by real-world challenges faced by families and caregivers, missed warning signs, preventable emergencies and systems that intervene too late. These experiences fueled her commitment to building intelligent solutions that preserve independence, reduce avoidable harm and restore peace of mind.

With more than 25 years of experience across pharmaceuticals, healthcare, business and technology, Corlette is a sought-after speaker and advocate for smarter care models. She is the inventor of care-focused technologies and a recipient of an international business award recognizing her impact and leadership. Grounded in the belief that technology must serve humanity, not replace it, her work bridges compassion with innovation.

In **The Care Code**, Corlette offers both a call to action and a practical roadmap for families, caregivers and health systems ready to care earlier, smarter and more intentionally, before crisis becomes the norm.

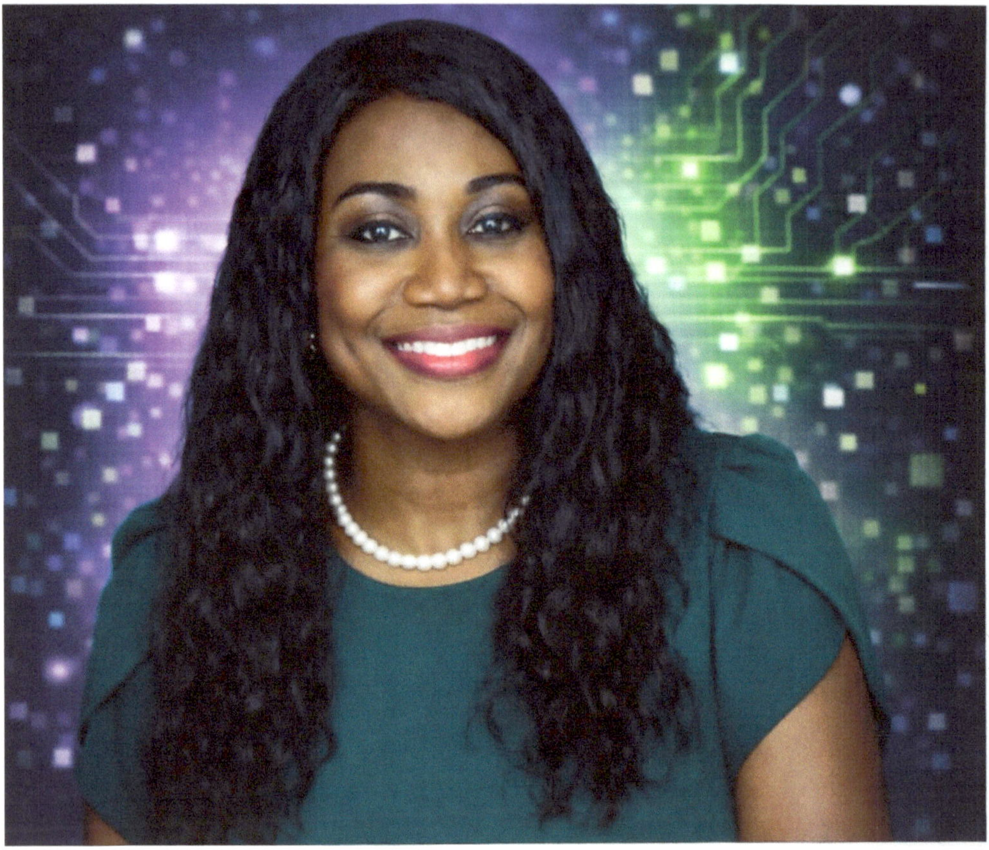

Sources

Centers for Disease Control and Prevention. (2023). *Chronic disease overview.* https://www.cdc.gov/chronicdisease/index.htm

Centers for Disease Control and Prevention. (2024). *Important facts about falls.* https://www.cdc.gov/falls/data-research/facts-stats/index.html

Centers for Disease Control and Prevention, National Institute for Occupational Safety and Health. (2024). *Healthcare worker well-being.* https://www.cdc.gov/niosh/healthcare/impactwellbeing/professional-wellbeing.html

Centers for Medicare & Medicaid Services. (2024). *National health expenditure data.* https://www.cms.gov/data-research/statistics-trends-and-reports/national-health-expenditure-data

Deloitte. (2025). *Future of health: Proactive and preventive care models.* https://www.deloitte.com/global/en/Industries/life-sciences-health-care.html

Journal of Medical Internet Research. (2023). *Remote patient monitoring and emergency utilization.* https://www.jmir.org/

MyDecine. (2024). *Preventive care vs. reactive care.* https://mydecine.com/preventive-care-vs-reactive-care-choose-health-save-money-and-live-longer/

National Center on Caregiving. (2024). *Family caregiver statistics and economic impact.* https://www.nccdp.org/family-caregiver-strain-and-the-hidden-economy-of-care/

National Institutes of Health. (2009). *Medication adherence and falls among older adults.* https://pmc.ncbi.nlm.nih.gov/articles/PMC2854886/

PubMed. (2010). *Medication adherence and fall risk in older adults.* https://pubmed.ncbi.nlm.nih.gov/27150680/

Remington Report. (2024). *Remote patient monitoring cost savings and readmission reductions.* https://remingtonreport.com/remote-patient-monitoring-the-cost-savings-and-readmission-reductions-for-specific-medical-conditions-in-home-care/

Rm2.ai™. (2026). *Predictive health monitoring platform overview.* https://rm2.ai

United for ALICE. (2024). *Health care affordability and household stability.* https://www.unitedforalice.org/health-care

WiFi Talents. (2024). *AI in the senior care industry statistics.* https://wifitalents.com/ai-in-the-senior-care-industry-statistics/

World Health Organization. (2022). *Falls prevention in older age.* https://www.who.int/news-room/fact-sheets/detail/falls

World Health Organization. (2023). *Ageing and health.* https://www.who.int/news-room/fact-sheets/detail/ageing-and-health

arXiv. (2025). *Machine learning models for medication adherence and hospitalization risk.* https://arxiv.org/abs/2504.07422

Reference-to-Chapter

Introduction & Preface
CDC (2024); WHO (2023); PubMed (2010); NIH (2009)

Chapter 1 – Cracking the Code: Why Health Care Needs Innovation
CDC (2026); CDC (2024); CDC (2023); WHO (2003); WHO (2023); NIH (2009); PubMed (2010)

Chapter 2 – The AI Advantage
Journal of Medical Internet Research (2023); WiFi Talents (2024); Remington Report (2024)

Chapter 3 – Living Better, Not Just Longer
WHO (2023); Deloitte (2025); CMS (2024)

Chapter 4 – The Predictive Power of Data
JMIR (2023); Remington Report (2024); arXiv (2025)

Chapter 5 – Early Warnings Save Lives
CDC (2024); WHO (2022); JMIR (2023)

Chapter 6 – Empowerment for Caregivers
National Center on Caregiving (2024); United for ALICE (2024)

Chapter 7 – Caregiving Without Filters
No external citations required (narrative chapter)

Chapter 8 – Dignity, Independence, and Aging in Place
WHO (2023); CDC (2023)

Chapter 9 – Just Listen
No external citations required (narrative chapter)

Chapter 10 – The Financial Burden of Reactive Care
CMS (2024); Deloitte (2025); MyDecine (2024); CDC NIOSH (2024)

Chapter 11 – Reducing Healthcare Costs Through Prevention
CMS (2024); Deloitte (2025); Remington Report (2024)

Chapter 12 – The True Cost of Doing Nothing
National Center on Caregiving (2024); United for ALICE (2024); Remington Report (2024); arXiv (2025)

Final Chapters & Manifesto
Deloitte (2025); WHO (2023); CDC (2024)

Rm2.ai™

HEALTH INTELLIGENCE FOR LIFE™

Rm2.ai™

HEALTH INTELLIGENCE FOR LIFE

Want To Learn More? Scan The QR Code:

www.ingramcontent.com/pod-product-compliance
Ingram Content Group UK Ltd.
Pitfield, Milton Keynes, MK11 3LW, UK
UKHW060005051026
15591UKWH00001B/50
* 9 7 9 8 9 9 0 4 0 7 0 1 5 *